TO LIVE AND DIE IN AMERICA

The Future of World Capitalism
Series editors: Radhika Desai and Alan Freeman

The world is undergoing a major realignment. The 2008 financial crash and ensuing recession, China's unremitting economic advance, and the uprisings in the Middle East, are laying to rest all dreams of an 'American Century'. This key moment in history makes weighty intellectual demands on all who wish to understand and shape the future.

Theoretical debate has been derailed, and critical thinking stifled, by apologetic and superficial ideas with almost no explanatory value, 'globalization' being only the best known. Academic political economy has failed to anticipate the key events now shaping the world, and offers few useful insights on how to react to them.

The Future of World Capitalism series will foster intellectual renewal, restoring the radical heritage that gave us the international labour movement, the women's movement, classical Marxism, and the great revolutions of the twentieth century. It will unite them with new thinking inspired by modern struggles for civil rights, social justice, sustainability, and peace, giving theoretical expression to the voices of change of the twenty-first century.

Drawing on an international set of authors, and a world-wide readership, combining rigour with accessibility and relevance, this series will set a reference standard for critical publishing.

Also available:

Geopolitical Economy:
After US Hegemony, Globalization and Empire
Radhika Desai

The Birth of Capitalism:
A Twenty-First-Century Perspective
Henry Heller

Remaking Scarcity:
From Capitalist Inefficiency to Economic Democracy
Costas Panayotakis

To Live and Die in America

Class, Power, Health, and Healthcare

Robert Chernomas and Ian Hudson

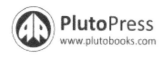
PlutoPress
www.plutobooks.com

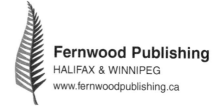
Fernwood Publishing
HALIFAX & WINNIPEG
www.fernwoodpublishing.ca

First published 2013 by Pluto Press, 45 Archway Road, London N6 5AA
www.plutobooks.com

Distributed in the United States of America exclusively by Palgrave Macmillan, a division of
St. Martin's Press LLC, 175 Fifth Avenue, New York, NY 10010

Published in Canada by Fernwood Publishing, 32 Oceanvista Lane, Black Point, Nova Scotia,
B0J 1B0 and 748 Broadway Avenue, Winnipeg, Manitoba, R3G 0X3
www.fernwoodpublishing.ca

Fernwood Publishing Company Limited gratefully acknowledges the financial support of the
Government of Canada through the Canada Book Fund and the Canada Council for the Arts, the
Nova Scotia Department of Communities, Culture and Heritage, the Manitoba Department of
Culture, Heritage and Tourism under the Manitoba Publishers Marketing Assistance Program
and the Province of Manitoba, through the Book Publishing Tax Credit, for our publishing
program.

   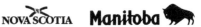

Library and Archives Canada Cataloguing in Publication
Chernomas, Robert
       To live and die in America : class, power, health and health care / Robert Chernomas, Ian
Hudson. (The future of world capitalism)
Includes bibliographical references.
ISBN 978-1-55266-561-9
       1. Medical economics--United States. 2. Medical care--United States. 3. Health status
indicators--United States. 4. Social classes--Health aspects--United States. 5. United States-
-Economic conditions--21st century. 6. United States--Social conditions--21st century.
I. Hudson, Ian, 1967- II. Title. III. Series: Future of world capitalism (Winnipeg, Man.)
RA410.53.C54 2013   362.10973   C2012-906999-X

British Library Cataloguing in Publication Data
A catalogue record for this book is available from the British Library

ISBN 978 0 7453 3217 8 Hardback
ISBN 978 0 7453 3212 3 Paperback
ISBN 978 1 55266 561 9 (Fernwood)
ISBN 978 1 8496 4842 4 PDF eBook
ISBN 978 1 8496 4844 8 Kindle eBook
ISBN 978 1 8496 4843 1 EPUB eBook

Library of Congress Cataloging in Publication Data applied for

This book is printed on paper suitable for recycling and made from fully managed and sustained
forest sources. Logging, pulping and manufacturing processes are expected to conform to the
environmental standards of the country of origin.

10 9 8 7 6 5 4 3 2 1

Designed and produced for Pluto Press by Curran Publishing Services, Norwich
Simultaneously printed digitally by CPI Antony Rowe, Chippenham, UK and
Edwards Bros in the United States of America

For my brother Fred. He would have understood;
he always did.

RC

For Brett and Mark, best brothers ever.

IH

CONTENTS

FIGURES AND TABLES

FIGURES

TABLES

ACKNOWLEDGMENTS

In writing this book we have been very fortunate to have benefited from the supportive people at Pluto Press. We owe a particular debt to Radhika Desai, co-editor of the Future of World Capitalism series, who went through both a fairly preliminary version and a much more polished draft with what could only be described as a fine toothcomb. Her thoughtful suggestions and insightful questions led to a much-improved version of the manuscript. The other co-editor, Alan Freeman, with the able assistance of Susan Dianne Brophy, has been particularly energetic on the publicity front, in an effort to ensure that this book actually gets read by more than a few people.

There have been a host of people at Pluto that have helped, in one important way or another, in getting the manuscript into actual finished book form. Our copy editor, Susan Curran, managed the impressive task of carefully eliminating our grammatical errors. Roger van Zwanenberg, David Shulman, Robert Webb, Jonathan Maunder and Melanie Patrick have all answered our enquiries about the ins and outs of publishing details, from image permissions to indexing, with great patience and good advice.

The manuscript also passed through the hands of anonymous reviewers who were reassuringly positive about the general direction of the research and also made some valuable suggestions for improvement. Finally, we received financial assistance for writing the book from the Global Political Economy Research Fund in the Faculty of Arts at the University of Manitoba, which we used to hire Rosa Sanchez, who did sterling work as a research assistant.

1

CLASS, POWER, HEALTH, AND HEALTHCARE

INTRODUCTION

In a 1974 speech to the First Conservative Political Action Conference, then Governor (and President to be) Ronald Reagan told a predictably receptive crowd that the United States was the greatest nation in the world. "Pope Pius XII said, 'Into the hands of America God has placed the destinies of an afflicted mankind.' We are indeed, and we are today, the last best hope of man on earth" (Reagan, 1974). This is one of the stronger statements of what is often called US exceptionalism—the idea that the United States is a unique and superior country. Unfortunately, in terms of the health of its people, the United States may be unique, at least among wealthy nations, but it is decidedly not superior.

This book is about how class and power in the United States have determined its health outcomes and healthcare system. The core argument is that disease and death in all nations, including the United States, are predominately structured and influenced by social and economic imperatives, not by irresistible laws of nature that are independent of socially determined political and economic factors (Cairns, 1971; Cassel, 1976; Chernomas, 1999; Chernomas and Donner, 2004; Dubos, 1959; 1965; Galdston, 1954; Navarro et al., 2003; Poland et al., 1998; Wilkinson, 1996). The specific evolution of US capitalism has shaped these social conditions and the healthcare system that evolved to deal with them. If class and power are the two most important determinants of everyday life in the United States, it follows that improving health in the United States will require a change in the system of power, and in turn the conditions in which people live and work, as well as a restructured healthcare system.

1

The United States has by far the most expensive healthcare system in the world, the worst health among wealthy industrialized nations by almost all measures, and is the only industrialized nation without some form of universal healthcare. US life expectancy is 79.6 years. According to the 2010 United Nations Human Development Index this places it behind 28 other countries, following Greece and Lichtenstein and just above Costa Rica, Portugal and Cuba. In terms of mortality rates for children under five, it ranks a worrying 46th just behind the UAE and above Chile (United Nations, 2011).

These results are not because of underfunding of the US healthcare system. The United States spends more in absolute and relative terms than any other industrial economy. In 2008, the United States spent 16 percent of its GDP on healthcare. This is the highest of the 31 countries in the Organisation for Economic Co-operation and Development (OECD) by a considerable margin. The second ranked country, France, spent 11 percent and the OECD average was a much more modest 9 percent. The combined level of public and private healthcare spending per person is also much higher in the United States than any other country. The United States spent $7,500 per person, while the second highest nation, Norway, spent only $5,000 (OECD, 2010). The disparity between healthcare spending and health outcomes suggests that the United States has a particularly inefficient healthcare system, but this divergence is also driven by social and economic conditions that create a less healthy US population.

In the context of these discouraging health indicators, the United States has recently been through a national debate on the future of its healthcare system. President Obama made universal access to healthcare an important plank in his 2008 election campaign. As we will show in Chapter 5, while Obama did manage to expand access, this was accomplished in a manner that maintained many of the features of the US system that contribute to its higher costs and poorer outcomes.

It is critical to point out, however, that not all capitalist nations have the same class and power relations, and therefore we should expect them to have different health outcomes and qualitatively different healthcare systems. One famous typology of capitalist nations groups countries into four categories (extended from Esping-Anderson's (1990) original three groups). Social democratic welfare states (like Sweden), are egalitarian (including more equal access to healthcare), and have strong protective regulations like environmental laws. In these nations, historically strong labor movements and other civil actors have been able to challenge the power of business and successfully develop a broad network of policies that alleviate, to a certain extent, many of the conditions that give rise to poor health outcomes in modern capitalism (Olsen, 2011: 4–6). The second group of nations is conservative-corporatist welfare states, which tend to provide relatively generous health and social services based on union membership or religious affiliation (like Italy). The third category—wage earner welfare states—provide limited benefits based on employment rather than being universal (like Australia). Finally, liberal welfare states contain a minimum safety net, offering basic social and health services to the poorest and elderly (like the United States). These countries have a history of relatively weak labor organizations and other social movements relative to the power wielded by the business community. This has resulted in a political and economic system with greater inequality and less regulatory intervention (Olsen, 2011: 4–6).

In an international health context, the liberal welfare state embraced by the United States should be viewed as a cautionary tale. As a result of the ability of social democratic countries to win redistributive policies, including an egalitarian healthcare system, and regulatory checks on business activities, people in these countries have superior health results (like lower infant mortality) than other nations (Navarro et al., 2003; Raphael and Bryant, 2004; Birn, Pillay, and Holtz, 2009). The wide variation of political and economic structures that exist between the social democratic and liberal nations suggests that, while the capitalist system does have inherent trends, there is still considerable scope for class politics—the conflict and collaboration of classes and groups—in each country to alter the conditions that create health problems, the health systems that deal with them and their outcomes.

COMPETING THEORIES OF HEALTH OUTCOMES

The emphasis in the preceding section on economic and social factors might come as something of a surprise to readers. Probably the dominant approach to understanding illness is the biomedical approach, in which the causes of disease stem from germs and genes. These illnesses are governed by natural and medical "laws." The treatment strategy that follows from this theory of disease is preoccupied with the search for bad genes, viruses, and bacteria. Treatments are focused on restructuring the biology of the individual through surgery, genetic intervention, or pharmaceuticals. To use an analogy, the biomedical approach views human health in much the same way that a mechanic would view a car. Individual components that are not working correctly need to be repaired or replaced. The biomedical approach can certainly boast an impressive list of scientific innovations that cure a very wide swath of illnesses. Medical innovations have also resulted in preventive measures like vaccinations. Yet, as we shall explain in Chapter 2, the biomedical approach cannot claim the credit for diagnosing the principal causes of, or providing the solution for, the major diseases of the nineteenth and twentieth centuries.

A second popular model explains health outcomes through individual lifestyle choices. According to the behavioral approach, the solution is to eliminate these self-destructive preferences. There is an important element of truth in this claim. If people don't smoke, there is less chance that they will get lung cancer. If people eat their vegetables and exercise regularly, they have less chance of heart disease. As we will show later in the chapter, however, there are several important shortcomings with this emphasis on the individual. The first is that people in different social situations but with identical lifestyle choices have different health results. The second is that it fails to explain why individuals make these choices. This is especially important since many supposedly individual choices appear to be heavily influenced by social position. If choices are genuinely individual, they should be evenly distributed across different groups in society, but they are not. People from lower socio-economic status have less nutritious diets, smoke more, and exercise less than do those from higher up the social ladder (Lantz et al., 1998; Nettle, 2010). In fact, many health problems are less a result of individual choice than they are a product of social circumstance rooted in the class-based circumstances and opportunities described throughout this book.

In stressing the importance of the political and economic environment in determining human health, we are advocating a political economy approach. According to this view, the way in which the economy operates, an individual's place in it, and in the social and political systems that go with it, have a strong influence on health outcomes. Of particular importance, in this view, are the power relationships that exist in a society. In our society power is largely conferred through ownership (especially, as Karl Marx famously noted, of the productive capacity). So the people who own firms have more power than their employees. Economic, political and social systems play an important role in determining both the environment in which people live and their ability to access the resources (things like food, shelter and medical care) necessary to enjoy a healthy life. In the words of a leading textbook on international health, "a political economy of health approach uncovers how personal, household, social, political, and economic conditions interrelate at various levels to produce particular health circumstances and outcomes" (Birn et al., 2009: 140). This is not to suggest that the biomedical and behavioral approaches are entirely incorrect. Rather, by placing biomedical and behavioral factors in their larger context, the political economy approach allows for a more complete explanation of human health.

An example might help illustrate the difference between the three approaches. When Andrea Martin was 42 years old she was diagnosed with an advanced case of breast cancer. After aggressive treatment, cancer was found in her other breast, and later still, she was found to have a large malignant brain tumor from which she died. Martin was also one of the volunteer subjects in a study that measured the "body burden" of chemicals in people. Biomonitoring by the Center for Disease Control (CDC), led by researchers from Mt. Sinai School of Medicine in 2003, revealed that Martin had at least 95 toxic chemicals in her system, 59 of which were cancer causing. Martin said at the time, "I was shocked at the breadth and variety of the number of chemicals. I was outraged to find out that without my permission, without my knowledge, my body was accumulating this toxic mixture" (Malkan, 2003). It is not as though Martin had a lifestyle that would make her more likely to come into contact with more chemicals than the average person. She did not work in a lab or at a nuclear reactor. The chemicals in her body were accumulated in the common acts of consuming everyday products and living a very average life in California. That an average life involves absorbing a large number of dangerous chemicals should perhaps not come as a complete surprise. The Registration, Evaluation, and Authorization of Chemicals (REACH) program of the European Union estimates that over the last 50 years over 75,000 new chemicals have been released into the environment.

The biomedical approach would have searched for Andrea Martin's genetic propensity for cancer, the results of her breast cancer screening, and then extolled the benefits of the chemotherapeutic and surgical treatment options available to treat her disease. The behavioral approach would have encouraged Martin to avoid food, air, and water contaminated with carcinogens. The political economy approach would suggest that she had limited control over, and little information about, the conditions under which she made her choices, which are driven by broader political and economic forces. Obviously, these different approaches are not completely exclusive. Genetics, behaviors, and political economic conditions most certainly all play a role in health outcomes. Yet the argument in this book is that they are not all equally important. In the battle for resources, where tradeoffs exist in how we choose to tackle health issues, the biomedical and behavioral approaches currently receive far too much prominence at the expense of the more effective political economy approach.

While this book is certainly within the political economy tradition, it attempts to delve deeper: just what is it that creates the social and economic conditions that, according to the political economy perspective, influence health outcomes so profoundly? So, while the political economy approach examines how inequality or environmental factors influence health, we will put forward a theory about what creates these problems. In its very condensed form, the argument is that political and economic results like pollution, working conditions and inequality are determined in large part by the twin dynamics of the capitalist economy—competition between firms and class conflict. Businesses in a capitalist economy must continuously strive to maximize profits in order to compete successfully with their rivals. However, the conditions under which firms maximize profits, from the wages they offer to the pollution that they emit, are the result of an ongoing social and political conflict over the rules of the capitalist game among business, on the one hand, and the "working class," which is so often harmed by these actions, on the other. (The question of just what constitutes the working class has been the subject of much debate, but we will associate workers with Lester Thurow's nonsupervisory workers, "those who don't boss anyone else—a vast majority of the workforce" (Thurow, 1996: 2), which according to the Bureau of Labor Statistics made up 82.5 percent of all employees in the United States in December of 2011 (Bureau of Labor Statistics, 2012: 8).) The dual dynamics of profitability and conflict can explain both the political economic results in specific capitalist countries that influence health and why the United States has such a unique healthcare system.

THE REST OF THE BOOK

This book examines how economic developments and class forces in the United States have contributed to the conditions that impact human health and to the evolution of the healthcare system that attempts to deal with its effects.

Chapter 2 challenges the conventional biomedical view of what is called the "epidemiological transition." Whereas the population generally died of infectious disease in the nineteenth century, the twentieth century was dominated by chronic disease. The popular understanding of this transition is that the germs that caused infectious disease mortality were defeated by the "magic bullets" of mainstream medicine, permitting the population to grow old enough to get heart disease and cancer. This is unambiguously false. The biomedical approach did not provide the solution for infectious disease, and neither biomedical nor behavioral approaches have been successful in explaining the rise in chronic disease or very effective at curing it.

Chapter 3 examines the US experience with respect to the infectious disease stage of capitalist development, to provide an alternative explanation of the epidemiological transition. We argue that early capitalism resulted in workers and their families being underfed and overworked, inhibiting their inborn and acquired immune system from working effectively, creating an "epidemic constitution" for infectious disease. The chapter focuses on the working and living conditions in the United States that created the infectious disease epidemic constitution, and the struggle for higher wages, occupational safety, child labor laws, the eight-hour day and public health measures that proved to be the solution. It will establish that class struggle was the key determinant of health in the epidemiological transition in the United States.

In Chapter 4, health in the more recent, affluent stage in the United States is examined. When workers successfully managed to improve their living standards, capitalists had to respond by moving to techniques that increased productivity so that rising wage costs and taxes could be accommodated without long-term threats to profits. The resulting mechanization and chemicalization of production created an epidemic constitution for chronic disease. This chapter will focus on the qualitative changes to the goods we consume, the environment that we live in, the conditions in which we work, and degree of equality, to explain the major killers of the population. Without dramatic social and economic changes, health results in the United States will continue to lag behind those in the rest of the world.

Chapter 5 switches the focus from the broader social context for health to examine the narrower field of the political economics of healthcare. Healthcare focuses on the production and distribution of specific goods and services that are seen as being directly related to health status (Evans, 1984: 3). A careful analysis of the specific characteristics of healthcare has led many economists to question the efficiency of a market-based healthcare system. Yet more than any other country in the industrialized world, the United States has implemented a market-based healthcare system. The evolution of the inferior US healthcare system can be explained with the same political economy tools that were used to analyze the problematic social conditions that influence US health. After the Second World War, citizens in other industrial countries demanded and received various forms of universal healthcare, while similar attempts in the United States were defeated because of a concerted effort by its capitalist class. Opposition to universal healthcare culminated in the contradictory Obama reforms, where a specific subsection of US business—what we later refer to as the medical industrial complex—triumphed at the expense of other US firms, and the majority of US citizens.

Chapter 6 draws from the examples set by the rest of the world to demonstrate that even within a capitalist economy, dramatic improvements can be made in the social and economic conditions that currently plague the United States. The twin problems of inefficient healthcare and a harmful economic, social, and physical environment require far-ranging changes to US public policy, which would only be possible with a vast restructuring of class relationships. However, just this kind of change has been made in different jurisdictions, when working people have organized effectively to demand it. We will look at three changes that could dramatically improve health results in the United States: the European Union's REACH legislation, altering the conditions of work and income distribution to improve the social conditions that are important to health, and a universal, single-payer, not-for-profit publicly administered healthcare system.

To get started we turn to the dramatic changes in life expectancy over the past 150 years.

2

THE MEDICAL MIRACLE?

There I am standing by the shore of a swiftly flowing river and I hear the cry of a drowning man. So I jump into the river, put my arms around him, pull him to shore and apply artificial respiration, and then just as he begins to breathe, another cry for help. So back in the river again, reaching, pulling, applying, breathing and then another yell. Again and again, without end, goes the sequence. You know, I am so busy jumping in, pulling them to shore, applying artificial respiration, that I have no time to see who the hell is pushing them all in.

(K. Zola, "Helping—does it matter: the problems and prospects of mutual aid groups," Address to the United Ostomy Association, 1970)

Dying isn't as easy as it used to be. From the onset of the industrial revolution until fairly recently, it was something of an accomplishment to live through childhood. Even when people made it through the deadly childhood years, there were a host of infectious diseases waiting to strike them down. In the last 150 years or so, there has been a remarkable transformation in both the life expectancy of the population of the industrialized world and the manner in which people die. The conventional understanding of this transformation is one of biomedical triumph. According to this theory, infectious diseases were conquered as medical science developed cures and vaccines. The reduction in infectious diseases allowed people to live long enough to fall prey to the chronic illnesses of heart disease and cancer, which are the major causes of death today. The biomedical approach should therefore be employed against the current killers in order to repeat its successes against infectious disease (Sargent, 2005; for a thorough review and critique of this literature see Porter, Ogden and Pronyk, 1999; Krieger, 2011: 131–6). The only problem with this version of history is that it is not true.

ILLNESS UNDER EARLY INDUSTRIALIZATION IN THE
UNITED STATES AND THE UNITED KINGDOM

In the nineteenth century people generally died of infectious diseases like tuberculosis, and their life expectancy was shockingly short—often less than 40 years. Figures 2.1 and 2.2 show the major causes of death in England and Wales (which as part of the first industrialized nation were trailblazers in terms of disease and economic trends) and the United States respectively. In England and Wales almost 50 percent of the deaths were caused by what could broadly be defined as infectious disease. Infectious disease was an even larger proportional killer in urban centres. In London 55 percent of deaths were caused by infectious disease, in Salford 58 percent, and in the notoriously insanitary central Liverpool 60 percent (Mooney, 2007: 600–1). As Figure 2.2 shows, the two leading causes of death in the United States were pneumonia and tuberculosis. Total infectious

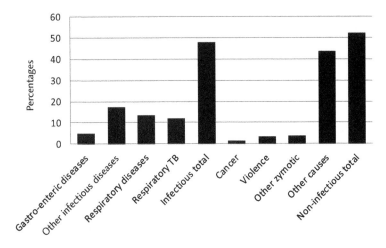

Figure 2.1 Causes of death in England and Wales, 1851–60

Cause groups include the following:
Gastro-enteric: cholera, diarrhoea and dysentery.
Other infectious: smallpox, measles, scarlatina, diphtheria,whooping cough, typhus, scrofula, tabes, mesenterica, hydrocephalus.
Respiratory diseases: bronchitis, laryngitis, pleurisy, pneumonia, asthma.
Respiratory TB: phthisis, consumption, pulmonary, tuberculosis.
Other causes: diseases of heart, brain, stomach, kidneys, generative organs, joints, and skin, childbirth, all other causes.
Column totals do not always sum to 100 percent because of rounding.

Source: from Money (2007: Table 1, p. 600), calculated from Registrar-General's Decennial Supplements, 1851–60.

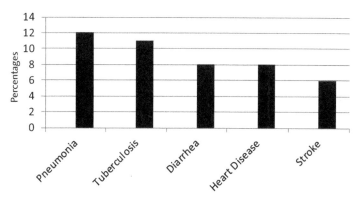

Figure 2.2 Leading causes of death in the United States, 1900

Source: National Center for Health Statistics (2006).

diseases are the largest category in what Birn and colleagues classify as "diseases of marginalization and deprivation" (2009: 266). While not all of the diseases in this category are infectious (death in childbirth, for example, is not even a disease), most of the non-infectious causes of illness and death were due to the same factors, and alleviated by the same remedies, that we describe for infectious disease in this chapter. We shall therefore use infectious disease as a shorthand term for this larger category.

Starting in England, and spreading to the other industrializing nations, people stopped dying young in such large numbers as the incidence of infectious disease declined. Figure 2.3 shows the increase in life expectancy in the United Kingdom and the United States. In the United Kingdom, life expectancy started to increase rapidly in the last half of the 1800s. Though starting from a higher level, the United States experienced a decline in life expectancy between 1800 and 1850 which has been called the "antebellum paradox." People during this period were also smaller in stature, further indicating some deterioration of health. Although a number of reasonable hypotheses have been suggested to explain this deterioration— including poorer nutrition, increased incidence of disease and greater urbanization—historians have not arrived at a consensus on the cause (Hacker, 2010: 53). After 1900, however, US trends caught up with those in the United Kingdom and remained similar. At any point in time, a similar relationship can also be demonstrated by taking cross-sectional data from countries at different levels of income. Figure 2.4 plots countries by their gross domestic product

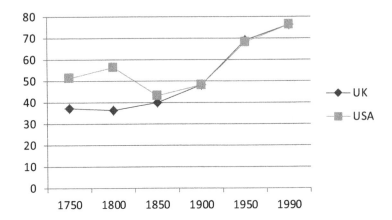

Figure 2.3 Life expectancy at birth in the United Kingdom and United States, 1750 to 1900

Source: Fogel (2004, Table 1.1.2).

(GDP) and life expectancy, producing a shape known as the Preston curve. Notice that in the Preston curve, at lower levels of income, small income gains lead to much larger increases in life expectancy than they do at higher levels of income. The broad conclusion is

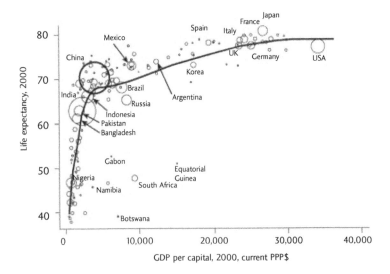

Figure 2.4 The Preston curve: life expectancy versus GDP per capita, 2000

Source: Cutler et al. (2006, Figure 1, 98).

inescapable. As incomes increase, people die later. This is in many ways a story of triumph. An increase in longevity means that fewer people suffer the tragedy of dying young from infectious disease. But who or what should get credit for this genuinely remarkable achievement?

The conventional story is that medical advance that prevented infectious disease was the primary savior. Proponents of the medical model argue that this great victory was achieved as germ after germ was isolated, the appropriate drug was developed and these diseases were inoculated out of existence. The triumph of medical science over debilitating illness has formed the basis for much of our understanding of how to identify and treat poor health in our society.

The idea that medical cures were responsible for improvement in human health was most famously, and successfully, challenged by Thomas McKeown (1976a). McKeown argued that the transition away from infectious disease and towards decreased mortality was not due to either medical advance or public health. The single determining factor was broad-based income gains for people and the corresponding increase in nutrition. McKeown's research was supported by Nobel Prize winning economic historian Robert Fogel (1997, 2004). Fogel (1997) examined the historical records on diet and height—on the assumption that people with better nutrition are larger—and concluded that practically the entire reduction in mortality during the 1800s was due to improved nutrition.

Few scholars question the validity of the "medical science played an insignificant role" portion of the McKeown thesis. It is true that the development of effective medical therapies further reduced mortality from infectious disease. But the historical record also makes it clear that the bulk of the reduction in infectious diseases occurred *before* mainstream medicine had developed its immunizations and antibiotics (Evans, Morris, and Marmor, 1994; McKeown, 1976a, 1979; McKinlay and McKinlay, 1977; Szreter, 2002a, 2003, 2004a, 2004b).   Figure 2.5 breaks down McKeown's original estimates of how much of the reduction in such disease happened after treatment for infectious disease was introduced in England and Wales. Only 25 percent of the mortality reduction in bronchitis, influenza, and pneumonia between 1901 and 1971 happened after treatment was introduced in 1938. For tuberculosis, only 33 percent of the mortality reduction happened after the 1947 introduction of treatment. McKeown himself argued that using data starting in 1900 would exaggerate the impact from

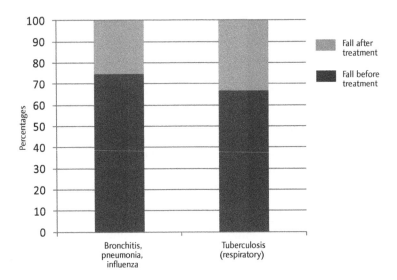

Figure 2.5 Fall in mortality from infectious diseases before and after introduction of treatment measures, England and Wales, 1901 to 1971

Source: McKeown et al. (1975, Table 9, p. 409).

the introduction of treatment, since a great deal of the decline in that disease happened in the latter decades of the nineteenth century (McKeown and Record, 1962: 104). As was the case with the United Kingdom, much of the mortality improvement in the United States was the result of the decreased number of fatalities from infectious diseases.

Figure 2.6 shows that the remarkable decline in eight infectious diseases in the United States came largely between 1900 and 1940. It also includes the date on which vaccination programs were introduced. As was the case with the United Kingdom, much of the reduction in these diseases predated the vaccination. Although the precise numbers in McKeown's original research have been criticized and qualified by subsequent authors (Wrigley and Schofield, 1981; Szreter, 1988), his overarching conclusion on the lack of connection between mortality and medical cures could not be challenged. In fact, it has been reinforced by more recent research. After surveying the existing literature on the subject, three prominent economists concluded that reductions in infectious disease (besides tuberculosis) from medical cures accounted for "only 3 percent of

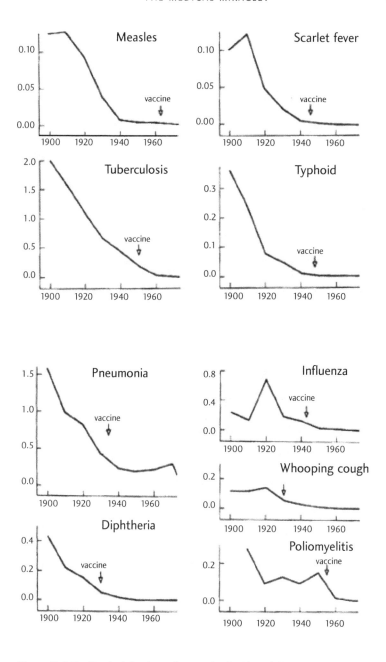

Figure 2.6 Decline in infectious diseases in the United States, 1900 to 1960

Source: McKinley and McKinley (1977: 422).

the total mortality reduction" (Cutler, Deaton, and Lleras-Muney, 2006: 103). In the now-developed world in general, reductions in tuberculosis mortality from medical cures accounted for another 10 percent, but this was not true of the United States, where the tuberculosis vaccine has never been used routinely, and Britain, where it was used "but without any evidence of an effect on trend mortality" (Cutler et al., 2006: 102).

Part of the reason for the lack of impact of vaccines is that evidence suggests that there is no inevitable connection between exposure to infectious disease and negative health impacts. Even in the late 1940s most adults in the United Kingdom were exposed to the TB bacillus. Unlike their ancestors few of them developed the disease, and fewer died. At present, one third of the world's population is infected with the TB bacillus, but only 5 to 10 percent of them become sick as a result (WHO, 2010). Most microorganisms are commonly harbored by the body with no ill effect. However, these same microbiota under "special conditions" exert a wide range of pathological effects. Those pathogens, usually considered to be disease producing, in all probability live consistently inside the human host without ill effects (Dubos, 1965).

It is generally agreed that medical interventions did not contribute substantially to health improvements in this period, but the McKeown/Fogel dismissal of broader public health measures has been challenged more successfully as a "dangerous untruth" (Szreter, 2002a: 722). The early 1900s saw a host of infrastructure projects such as sewage systems, fresh drinking water and draining swamps, which are what most people associate with public health, as well as broader social measures to improve the working and living conditions of the general public—from a social welfare system to rules on occupational safety and health. A number of researchers have pointed to different sources of evidence that all suggest that public health, broadly defined, played an important role. In his sympathetic re-examination of the McKeown thesis, James Colgrove (2002) cites two studies that show that specific public health interventions—improvements in milk and water quality in Philadelphia, and quarantine of infected people—had a large impact on infectious disease. Other authors have argued that while improved nutrition did play an important role in the decline in mortality from 1860 to 1950, widespread sanitary engineering and housing construction were also crucial (Brenner, 2005: 1215). Szreter claimed that the problem with McKeown's interpretation was that it "failed to emphasize the simultaneous historical importance of an accompanying redistributive social philosophy and practical politics, which has characterized the public health movement from its 19th-century origins" (Szreter, 2002a: 722).

Thus expanded to include the contribution of public health measures, McKeown's dismissal of the medical profession's claim to have vanquished infectious disease with scientific cures has stood the test of time—and considerable scrutiny. As we shall argue, all of these changes, from increased incomes for the populace, to improved sanitation to public health programs, were the result of hard-won gains by working people in both the economic and political realms. The point here is that it was improvements in the condition in which people live, rather than medical treatment of the symptoms of those wretched conditions, that cured the infectious disease epidemic.

This conclusion is bolstered from an unexpected source. An interesting natural experiment took place between 1955 and 1960. The Navaho-Cornell Field Health Research Project attempted to correct for the below-average health of residents of the Navaho native American reservation by bringing in modern medical services. This ambitious project provided a well-equipped ambulatory care facility, physicians, nurses, trained Navaho health aides, and transportation for hospital care. However, it was provided without changing the impoverished social and economic conditions of the residents, who were living in windowless, one-room log-and-mud dwellings with dirt floors, and had alarming rates of illiteracy and endemic poverty.

By objective criteria the project had some successes to report— some common problems among the Navahos, like ear infections among children, were sharply reduced. However, at the end of five years there was virtually no change in the overall disease pattern, and little, if any, change in the death rates, including a shockingly high infant mortality rate which persisted at three times the national average. The investigators concluded that the disease and mortality patterns of the Navaho were a result of the way they lived and could not be changed until basic changes took place in the tribe's way of life (Cassel, 1976: 71–2).

MODERN ILLNESS

People in industrialized capitalist countries do not die the way they used to. Between 1900 and 1940 in the United States, infectious disease, with its characteristic pattern, etiology, and duration, gave way to new and frequently more chronic forms of pathology and epidemic. Chronic disease is characterized by a slow development of disease and a long morbidity process, although this is not always apparent to the victim. As the incidence of mortality from infectious disease declined, heart disease and cancer became the new killers. A large increase in heart disease, for example, occurred between 1900 and 1960 (Blumenfeld, 1964; Brierley, 1970; Cairns, 1971; Galdston, 1954). In England and Wales in 2003, cardiovascular disease and cancer alone accounted for over 50 percent of all deaths (Figure 2.7). The same killers take the most lives in the United States (Figure 2.8).

The cancer statistics are stark. At the beginning of the twenty-first

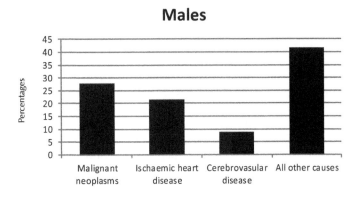

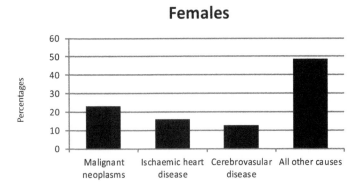

Figure 2.7 Causes of deaths for males and females in the United Kingdom, 2003

Source: Griffiths, Rooney, and Brock (2005: 4).

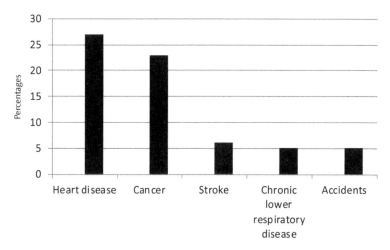

Figure 2.8 Leading causes of death in the United States, 2004

Source: National Center for Health Statistics (2006).

century half of the men and one third of the women will get cancer at some point in their life. In 2004 alone, 1.3 million people in the United States were diagnosed with cancer and over 500,000 were killed by it. Although there are many different types of cancer, the majority of deaths in the United States are caused by a surprisingly narrow range of killers. For men the big threats are lung and bronchus (32 percent), prostrate (10 percent), and colon and rectum (10 percent). For women it is lung and bronchus (25 percent), breast (15 percent), and colon and rectum (10 percent) (Faguet, 2005: 5, 8). Rates are not only high, but are also increasing. In the last half of the twentieth century the incidence (age adjusted and population adjusted) of cancer increased by 89 percent (Faguet, 2005: 13). Heart disease also became a major killer during this period. In 1900, heart disease only caused 8 percent of all deaths in the United States. Despite recent declines in heart disease (which are discussed in more detail in Chapter 4), by 2004 it was still responsible for 27 percent of deaths (Figures 2.2 and 2.8).

This transformation in the causes of death has come alongside advances in medical science. One possible explanation for the increase in cancers and heart disease is that these illnesses were present in earlier times but they could not adequately be detected by the more primitive diagnostic tools of the nineteenth century.

However, the ability to differentiate between heart disease and tumors on the one hand, and cholera and measles on the other, was well within the capabilities of the pathologists of the time. By the 1930s, the state of medical knowledge on cancer was surprisingly advanced (Davis, 2007: x, 20).

The increase in mortality from chronic disease has also occurred alongside an increase in life expectancy. It is possible that people were finally living long enough to acquire chronic disease. Yet there are problems with this explanation as well. It is true that in the early twentieth century, life expectancy in the industrialized capitalist countries was much lower than it is currently. However, these numbers exaggerate the real improvement in the life expectancy of adults. Figure 2.9 shows the life expectancy for people of different ages over time in the United Kingdom. Much of the increase in life expectancy is accounted for by the dramatic decrease in infant mortality that took place during that period, as opposed to adults actually living longer. In the 1850s, 45-year-olds would live to be 70 on average.

The same trend occurred in the United States, although slightly later. In Philadelphia in 1870, 175 out of 1,000 children born would not live to their first birthday, by 1900 this had improved slightly to 136 and by 1930 it had fallen considerably to 75 (Condran,

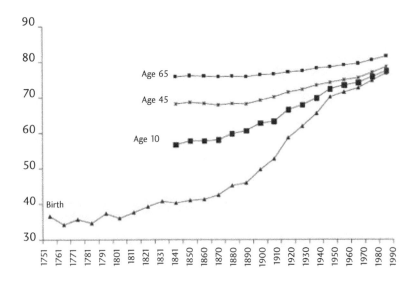

Figure 2.9 Expected age at death, England and Wales, 1751 to 1990

Source: Cutler et al. (2006: 100).

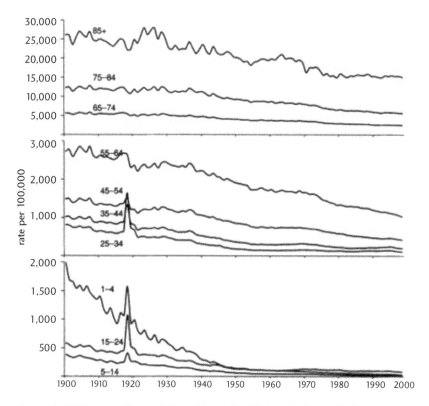

Figure 2.10 Age-specific mortality in the United States, 1900 to 2000

Source: Lynch et al. (2004, Fig 2, p. 360); data from National Center for Health Statistics.

Williams, and Cheney, 1997: 453). Figure 2.10 shows the decline of mortality by age group in the United States (the spike represents the influenza outbreak of 1918). The big decline in the early part of the twentieth century was due to the tremendous improvement in life chances of children under 4 years old. So the raw life expectancy numbers are misleading when it comes to the conclusion that we are living dramatically longer. A better conclusion is that we are not dying young.

More children surviving childhood, rather than more people living longer, still means that the United States, like all societies where this is happening, has an aging population. The percentage of the total population over the age of 65 has increased from 4.1 percent in 1900 to 13 percent in 2010 (USAA, 2010). It is also true that living longer increases the chances of getting cancer. From 1994 to 1998 for all races and combining both sexes, the cancer incidence for 35 to 39-year-olds was 130 per 100,000. This rises to 574 in the 50 to 54-year-old population, and 2,500 for those between 80 and 84 (USNIH, 2009). So this is responsible for part of the rise in cancer rates.

Yet this explanation is not sufficient. Those who lived into their sixth, seventh, and eighth decades in the nineteenth century rarely died of cancer or heart disease (McKeown, 1976a, 1979; McKinlay, McKinlay, and Beaglehole, 1989; Evans, Morris, and Marmor, 1994). The age-standardized incidence of cancer accounts for changes that have occurred over time in the age distribution of the population by comparing rates in people of the same age. For example, it compares cancer incidence for 50-year-old women in 1950 and 2000 in order to detect changes in cancer rates for similar people of similar ages. From 1950 to 1998, in the United States the age-standardized incidence of cancer rose about 60 percent. Breast cancer has grown by 60 percent and prostate cancer by 200 percent. In the United States, childhood cancers have increased by 26 percent and are the number one killer of children, after accidents. Between 1992 and 1999 in the United States only the incidence of lung cancer in men has decreased. Predominantly non-smoking cancers have continued to increase, including malignant melanoma by 18 percent, leukemia by 18 percent, breast by 7 percent, kidney by 14 percent, bone and joint by 20 percent, and thyroid cancer by 22 percent (Epstein et al., 2002).

If the dramatic increase in rates of cancer and heart disease cannot be explained satisfactorily by either better diagnostic tools or people getting older, what has caused the increase?

THE MEDICAL DIAGNOSIS

Some call New Jersey the Cancer State because of all the chemical companies there, but in fact, the major factor is probably your genetic constitution .... Basically, inequality comes from our genes.

(James Watson, former Head of the Human Genome Project, quoted in Cooper, 1994: 326)

Some academics have argued that the biomedical approach has been primarily responsible for the (admittedly smaller) gains in longevity since 1950. One of the principal champions of the biomedical approach is Cutler. He argues that the biomedical approach has been responsible for identifying, isolating and treating these new causes of death. For example, he estimates that two-thirds of the reduction in mortality from cardiovascular disease is due to advances in medicine (Cutler et al., 2006: 104). Not content with ascribing a driving role to medical science, Cutler downplays the impact of income. "Over the broad sweep of history, improvements in health and income are both the consequence of new ideas and new technology, and one might or might not cause the other" (Cutler et al., 2006: 116). However, Cutler has failed to explain why these new diseases have become the primary killers of those in industrial societies. Nor can he explain why the United States, which is supposedly the technological leader, is a laggard in terms of broadly defined health indicators if medical advance is the overwhelming driver of decreases in mortality.

Cutler's technological optimism is not universally shared. In keeping with his emphasis on the importance of income and nutrition, Fogel argues that although modern medicine has made life much more "bearable" it has done nothing to improve mortality (Fogel, 2004: 103). There has, it is true, been a significant decline in heart disease mortality starting around 1970, but at most 25 percent of this decline can be attributed to the effectiveness of medical intervention. As was the case with infectious disease, it seems the drop in mortality rates from cardiovascular disease began before most of these modern techniques had been developed (Rachlis and Kushner, 1989: 169–70).

The medical model's attempt to find a cure for cancer has also not proved particularly impressive despite a financial commitment commensurate with the declaration of a "war on cancer." The US government alone has spent an astonishing $69 billion on cancer research over the last 40 years, and treatment costs for cancer run at about $100 billion every year (Davis, 2007: 10). Yet success has been very elusive. Except for a few rare types of cancer, medicine cannot claim any improvements in prognosis for patients with the most common forms of the disease. Guy Faguet's damning indictment of the progress in this war must give even the most optimistic proponents of the medical model cause for concern. According to Faguet, the history of cancer cures has been the repeated tale of promising trials, massive investment, limited benefits, and unforeseen complications as drugs like Interferon and Interleukin-2 failed to provide the miracle cure. The very best that could be claimed for these remedies is that they have been effective on a few low-incidence cancer types like in situ bladder cancer

(Faguet, 2005: 65; see also Rachlis and Kushner, 1989: 171). To make matters worse on the drug front, success rates are getting worse. Almost all of the drugs that have proven effective against cancers were developed before 1983 (Faguet, 2005: 74).

This is not for want of effort. In an attempt to demonstrate that potential therapies have a statistically significant impact on cancer, drug companies have invested in increasingly large, and therefore expensive, clinical trials. For example, the clinical trials on Tamoxifen, a potential treatment for breast cancer, had a sample size of over 13,000 women and cost $68 million. This study discovered that it did reduce the risk of breast cancer by 49 percent, but increased the risk of endometrial cancer by 150 percent (Faguet, 2005: 107). The reason that such large and expensive trials are needed, according to Faguet, is that the limited effectiveness of new drugs is rarely picked up by smaller sample sizes, resulting in new drugs on the market that are "statistically significant but clinically irrelevant" (Faguet, 2005: 106). Faguet's less than optimistic conclusion is that "despite the most assiduous and lengthy efforts by the largest number of researchers ever assembled to conquer a disease, most advanced cancers respond only marginally to cytotoxic chemotherapy drugs" (2005: 82–3).

The statistics also make for grim reading. Treatment is considered successful if it results in five years of disease-free survival. Even on this definition, only 2 percent of all cases in the United States with advanced or metastatic cancer were successfully treated using chemotherapy, or a combination of chemotherapy and irradiation or surgery. For the nine most frequent cancers, which make up 51 percent of total deaths from cancer, both incidence and mortality have been increasing (Faguet, 2005: 87). The lack of success in curing advanced stages of cancer has led to an emphasis on quality of life for the cancer patient, which is an admission that while current medical approaches cannot save people (Faguet, 2005: 89), they might make them a little more comfortable as they die.

There are also some important questions about the health benefits from genetic research, the new frontier in medical science. Migrant populations provide an interesting test of the complicated relationship between genes and the environment. If genes determine our health results, then relocating a specific bundle of genetics to a new environment should have no effect. Yet this is not the case. In an excellent example of these kinds of study, migrants from ethnic groups with low breast cancer rates in China, Japan, and the Philippines were studied after they moved to the western United

States. The genetic explanation would suggest that there is something different in the genes between these ethnic groups and those of the same ethnic groups born in the United States, that would account for the difference in cancer rates. It would also suggest that, since genes do not change rapidly as a result of a change in environment, the new immigrants should maintain their lower rates of cancer. However, rates of breast cancer in the Asian women in the study rose once they settled in the United States. Further, the longer the migrants remained in the United States, the greater their incidence of breast cancer (Ziegler et al., 1993). According to a recent survey, studies on migrant populations "have shown the dominant role of environmental factors in determining cancer risk" (Kolonel and Wilkens, 2006: 198). Similar tests have been conducted on the incidence of heart disease. One study of people of Japanese ancestry who lived in Japan, Hawaii, and California found that those who were more "Westernized in their culture and social relations" had a higher rate of coronary heart disease (Marmot and Mustard, 1994: 204). The inescapable conclusion of these studies is that when people move from one region to another, they take on the risk of heart disease or cancer of the region to which they have relocated (Frank et al., 2006: 15).

While genes do matter, the way in which they determine health outcomes is complex. Recently the field of epigenomics has found that genetic behavior does not rely only on the genes themselves, but depends on a wide variety of "triggers" that can alter what the gene will do. So identical genetic make-up can result in very different results depending on what triggers are encountered. For example, the genes of twins are functionally identical at a very young age, but as twins age, they grow further apart, so that later in life they are significantly biologically different (PBS, 2007). Therefore, what determines a person's health is a complex interaction between their genes and the epigenomic triggers that a person encounters through their lives. Further, it appears as though a large number of these triggers are found in our environment, and that they may be preventing genes from combating some of the leading causes of sickness and death. To provide just one example, nickel and chromium increase DNA methylation, which switches off genes and leads to cancer (Hileman, 2009).

Class also interacts with genes in a complicated manner. While genes can make people vulnerable to disease, this vulnerability can be "triggered" by conditions dependent on social factors that are so often influenced by class (such as diet or lack of self-esteem), which will determine the degree to which the population will suffer from the illness (Baird, 1994). This implies that DNA alone cannot be the "master programmer" but can only be understood in the broader context of the organism and the environment (social and physical) in which it operates (Krieger, 2011: 139). The manner in which the genome is explored and what is done with that information is likely to be the subject of considerable debate because of the link between genetics, the environment, and social position.

The behavioral approach also offers an explanation for the growing incidence of chronic disease. In 1977 John Knowles, the president of the Rockefeller Foundation, argued that neither the medical community nor the government should be primarily responsible for the health of the US populace. Rather, the responsibility lay with individual decisions. Marc Lalonde, Canada's minister of national health, argued that our narcissistic society was undoing progress toward better health through "indolence, the abuse of alcohol, tobacco and drugs, and eating habits that put the pleasing of the senses above the needs of the human body" (Birn, Pillay, and Holtz, 2009: 346). In this view, personal choices about smoking lead to lung cancer, drinking harms the liver, and dietary choices contribute to heart disease. In a simplified form, this approach argues that the increase in heart attacks is caused by over-consumption of unhealthy foods, and the solution is to cut down on the intake of Bacon McCheeseburgers. A more academic wording of the argument would be that "human behavior is the single, most important determinant in variations in health outcomes" (Satcher and Higginbotham, 2008: 401).

According to one estimate, lifestyle choices account for more than 40 percent of the variation in health outcomes between people, compared with unequal access to healthcare which accounts for 15 to 20 percent, disparities in the physical and social environment, which account for 20 to 25 percent, and genetics, which accounts for another 20 to 25 percent (Satcher and Higginbotham, 2008: 401). The remedy for poor health outcomes, according to this model, is obviously to change people's behavior. The United States, for example, launched the Action for Healthy Kids in schools to encourage healthy lifestyles of nutrition and fitness. For adults, the 100 Black Men Health Challenge took a group of professionals and encouraged them to change their life in three ways: first, increase exercise and fruit and vegetable intake; second, quit smoking; and third, regularly visit a primary care provider. This has been claimed as "one of the most successful interventions targeting African American men," with the original target group now using their personal changes as a model to mentor black youth (Satcher and Higginbotham, 2008: 402).

As we mentioned in the Introduction, there are a number of problems with this interpretation of health. If we take smoking as one obvious, harmful behavioral choice, it might help to highlight its limitations. Tobacco is not only toxic but also addictive, and addiction commonly commences around the age of 14 (Evans et al., 1994). Consequently, the presumption that users rationally and voluntarily "choose" smoking as a "lifestyle" is not wholly appropriate. Furthermore, that smoking behavior is very sharply graded by socio-economic class (the lower the class the more likely people are to be addicted to tobacco) further undercuts the argument that smoking represents an individual choice, and suggests instead that it is at least in part the product of social position. In other words, people make individual lifestyle decisions within a social context. Finally, even those in the higher social and occupational grades who do choose to smoke have fewer of the adverse effects of tobacco (Evans et al., 1994: 6, 44). With a qualification for the addiction part of the story, a virtually identical tale could be told for the supposedly lifestyle impacts of diet and exercise. Working long hours, not being able to afford childcare, and lack of access to facilities make people much less likely to choose exercise as part of their lifestyle.

We are not suggesting that humans do not make individual choices. Working-class people do get to choose whether to smoke or make the much more difficult decision to quit. However, Chapter 4 will demonstrate that this choice, and the health consequences of that choice, is heavily influenced by social and economic factors.

In stressing the limits of explanations based on lifestyles and medicine, we are very much siding with scholars like Nancy Krieger, who propose a broader model of health that attempts to encompass the interactions between behavior, medical, and social factors, called the ecosocial model (2005). One of the key tenets of this model is that people "literally embody their lived experience" (Krieger, 2011: 215). While, the ecosocial model acknowledges the connections between our "inner and outer" selves, it views "the primary causal arrow as leading from societal conditions to health status" (Krieger, 2011: 215, 235). Rather than focusing on individual social determinants of health, it also attempts to discover ways in which social factors, behaviors, and biology interact to produce specific outcomes.

Gender, class, and smoking

There was a time when men smoked more than women. In 1965 in the United States, 52 percent of men smoked compared with 34 percent of women. A decline in overall rates of smoking has been accompanied by a narrowing of the gender gap. In 2009, 24 percent of men and 18 percent of women smoked (American Lung Association, 2011: 19). While the once pronounced gender difference in smoking is diminishing, there is a socio-economic distribution to smoking. In 2009, 31 percent of those below the poverty line smoked compared with 19 percent above the poverty line. Of people with a high-school education, 25 percent smoke, those with a BA, 11 percent, and those with a graduate degree, 6 percent (CDC, 2010). This trend has not gone unnoticed by the tobacco industry. One study, examining the marketing tactics of the two largest US cigarette companies, discovered that they "consider 'working class' young adults to be a critical market segment to promote growth of key brands." The authors conclude that because the disparity in smoking is becoming more of a class than a gender issue, "tobacco control resources" need to be targeted more explicitly at "working class" women (Barbeau, Leavy-Sperounis, and Balbach, 2004).

The divergence between smoking rates among socio-economic groups is not unique to the United States. In the United Kingdom, smoking has "all but lost its male identity … but is emerging as a habit sustained within working class communities." Increased smoking is associated with the twin pressures of greater caring responsibilities and reduced resources (Graham, 1994). Smoking rates among women with more socio-economic advantages have fallen more drastically than among women from lower socio-economic categories in the United Kingdom, suggesting that one sure method of reducing smoking would be to "raise the living standards" of the latter group (Graham and Der, 1998).

What is being suggested here is that neither the biomedical nor the behavioral explanations for the current pattern of disease are robust. In isolation, they cannot explain the current patterns of disease, nor are their solutions likely to provide wide-ranging remedies, although of course they can help individual cases. What these explanations lack is an understanding of the conditions that foster modern disease.

Rudolf Virchow and the social determinants of health

German physician Rudolf Virchow's (1821–1902) medical discoveries were so extensive that he is known as the "Father of Modern Pathology." However, he was also a trailblazer in identifying how societal policies determine health. In 1848, Virchow was sent by the Berlin authorities to investigate the epidemic of typhus in Upper Silesia. His Report on the Typhus epidemic prevailing in Upper Silesia argued that lack of democracy, feudalism, and unfair tax policies in the province were the primary determinants of the inhabitants' poor living conditions, inadequate diet, and poor hygiene that fuelled the epidemic.

Virchow stated that *disease is not something personal and special, but only a manifestation of life under modified (pathological) conditions.* Arguing *Medicine is a social science and politics is nothing else but medicine on a large scale,* Virchow drew direct links between social conditions and health. He argued that improved health required recognition that *if medicine is to fulfil her great task, then she must enter the political and social life. Do we not always find the diseases of the populace traceable to defects in society?* (Virchow, 1848/1985).

The authorities were not happy with the report and Virchow was relieved of his government position. But he continued his pathology research within university settings and went on to a parallel career as a member of Berlin City Council and the Prussian Diet, where he focused on public health issues consistent with his Upper Silesia report. Virchow also bitterly opposed Otto Von Bismarck's plans for national rearmament and was challenged to a duel by said gentleman. Virchow declined participation.

Source: quoted from Raphael (2010: 4).

THE CORPORATE INFLUENCE ON MEDICAL SCIENCE

Despite the inability of the narrowly defined medical approach to claim credit for the decline in infectious disease or much progress in solving chronic disease, the medical industries have been very successful in convincing the public that in the battle for improved health, resources should be dedicated to discovering medical cures for disease rather than improving social conditions. Why has this happened?

It was certainly not due to a lack of intellectual debate during the early industrial stage of capitalism among different schools of disease theory and practice. There were a number of scientist-reformers in all the developing capitalist countries who were part of larger movements for which the solutions to health problems were seen as political as well as scientific. The movement to promote sanitation and hygiene was not just about picking up litter or eliminating the need for an inconvenient nosegay, but was an attempt to redress, in some measure, the abysmal conditions of the wretched and unhealthy slums in which an impoverished working class was forced to wheeze away its sickly existence (Galdston, 1954: 118). For these researchers, epidemics were not rooted in germs but in socio-economic and political reality, and the solution was to be found in policy reform.

One particularly dedicated example was Max von Pettenkofer. He felt that the role of science was not to solve the problems of disease in the laboratory, but rather to provide the scientific foundation for social action. He ingested cholera bacilli to demonstrate that it was not the germs in isolation but the conditions in which the germs were encountered that mattered. He obtained a culture freshly isolated from a fatal case of the epidemic raging in Hamburg, and on October 7, 1882, swallowed a large amount of it on an empty stomach, the acidity of which had been neutralized by drinking an adequate quantity of sodium carbonate—the very conditions thought to be most favorable for the establishment of the disease. The number of bacilli ingested by Pettenkofer was immensely greater than that taken under normal conditions of exposure, and yet he experienced no symptoms except "light diarrhea," although an enormous proliferation of the bacilli could be detected in the stools. Shortly thereafter, several of Pettenkofer's followers repeated the experiment on themselves with the same result. None of them doubted that the bacillus was the cause of cholera. Although it would be unlikely to pass a modern-day ethics review board, the experiment demonstrated that infectious epidemics are complex phenomena involving not only the micro-organisms but also the physiological state of the patient, the environment, the social structure of the community, and countless other unsuspected factors. The implantation of bacilli, like the planting of seed, does not necessarily ensure a growth (Dubos, 1950: 271–2).

Yet in the competition for resources, mainstream medicine successfully eliminated its more socially attuned competitors. As we have seen, the triumph of mainstream medicine was not a product of its clear scientific superiority. Rather, it can be argued that it was financed and encouraged by capitalists and the institutions representing their interests, in the hope that it could solve medical problems without disturbing the dominant economic and social relations.

At the turn of the century in the United States, the Rockefellers, Carnegies, Morgans, and Huntingtons began to spend millions of dollars on university medical schools and the evaluation of medical education in general, including state education boards (Burrow, 1977). The Rockefellers started the Rockefeller Institute for Medical Research in 1901 and the General Education Board, which supported medical schools, in 1903. They also donated money to medical schools that followed the medical, rather than the more social, model. Harvard received almost $3 million in gifts from philanthropists including Rockefeller and Morgan. This trend was continued in the next few decades at other universities like Cornell, Vanderbilt, and Chicago. The most important of these university investments was most likely Rockefeller's support of the Johns Hopkins Medical School. Under the leadership of William Welch, a devotee of a narrowly defined, biological approach to medicine, and funded generously by Rockefeller, Hopkins became a model for other medical schools in the country (Burrow, 1977).

Perhaps more importantly, the Carnegie Foundation financed a survey of medical schools in North America by Abraham Flexner (a layman and the brother of Simon Flexner, the director of the Rockefeller Institute for Medical Research). The Flexner report of 1910, the result of surveying 69 medical schools in what must have been a whirlwind 78 working days, reached the public almost immediately upon completion and resulted in many medical school closures. Particularly hard hit were the non-allopathic institutions, which were criticized for treating disease with dietary changes. The criticized schools attempted to fight back, questioning Flexner's intellectual authority and arguing that his impact could only come from the "unlimited access to the pocketbook of a millionaire." They charged Rockefeller and Carnegie interests with seeking to gain control over medical practice from the state to the federal level. "Greedy capital," which had made workers in the United States "victims of plunder," now hoped to subjugate medical institutions (Burrow, 1977: 43–5). However, the schools were fighting a losing battle.

As a result of the Flexner report, philanthropists began to tie their contributions to universities that offered the narrow medical model favored in the report. Further, state legislatures were successfully convinced to make university medical accreditation dependent on adopting the Flexner reforms. Despite the misgivings of presidents of major US universities, who viewed this practice as a "menace to the freedom of teaching" (Burrow, 1977: 46), only schools that received contributions could afford the legally enforced standards, which were established by foundation leadership. In this way the foundations eliminated competition from the health sector, and deprived the "irregular groups" of credit for pointing out deficiencies in orthodox medical practice. The result was that narrowly defined medicine became the dominant social tool for dealing with health problems, despite the lack of evidence to support its supposed victory over infectious disease.

The trend toward medical research and training that focused on narrow, individual explanations for health was reinforced during the cold war. According to Nancy Krieger, in the intimidating political context of the red menace, Senator Joseph McCarthy, and the House Committee on Un-American Activities, medical research that rejected analysis based on the individual and focused on broader social factors was accused of criticizing the United States's free market system. After McCarthy claimed that 500 members of the American Men of Science belonged to "communist fronts" in 1950, researchers in a wide variety of disciplines, including medicine, linked with these "subversive" ideas were denied funding or removed from their positions (Krieger, 2011: 145). The political environment in the 1950s strengthened the direction of medical science initiated by the corporate-influenced Flexner Report.

Corporate influence on the medical profession is not a relic of medicine's naïve past. The highly lucrative world of modern medicine creates an incentive for corporations to influence the profession. This has been documented on a number of levels. Doctors' choice of treatments can be influenced through a wide array of corporate gifts, from free pens to all-expenses-paid educational conferences in exotic locations (Angell, 2004; Chren, Landefeld, and Murray, 1989; Lexchin, 1993; Gagnon and Lexchin, 2008). In 1999, the drug industry (to which we return in much more detail in Chapter 5) spent between $8,000 and $13,000 per doctor on promotions aimed at physicians in the United States (Gerth and Stolberg, 2000). The influence of the corporate world in medical training also continues in the modern system. The drug industry has a sizeable presence in most medical schools, both at the institutional level, through donations, making presentations and putting on conferences, and at a more individual level, by paying for medical students' books and sponsoring dinners for them. The conclusion of one study is that "The pharmaceutical industry has a significant presence during residency training, has gained the overall acceptance of trainees, and appears to influence prescribing behavior" (Zipkin and Steinman, 2005).

The corporate world has also spent considerable sums influencing the state of scientific debate. This most frequently occurs when studies come to light that either question the effectiveness or uncover dangerous side-effects of specific treatments. Threatened with the loss of a lucrative market, the understandable course of action for any firm is to mount a "case for the defense" of their maligned product. The now standard industry practice under these circumstances is for the firm to hire researchers to cast doubt on the critical research in a number of ways. This technique was pioneered by the tobacco industry's effort to undermine scientific evidence linking smoking to cancer. First, the specific design of the offending study is criticized in an attempt to label it "junk" science. Second, counter-studies can be commissioned that present conflicting or inconclusive evidence. This is an especially attractive route since often the affiliation between the researcher and the corporate benefactor of the study is never revealed, creating a false veneer of impartiality. Finally, experts can be hired to testify in front of regulatory bodies about the limitations of the study (Pearce, 2008). The overarching goal of these techniques is to cast doubt on any negative findings so that the case can be made, with at least some degree of credibility, that further testing is required before any remedial actions, like taking the drug off the market, are taken.

The structure of health institutions and the dominant methods that influence the state of knowledge in the profession are not the result of impartial scientific advance, although this is undoubtedly part of the story. They are also influenced by an ongoing conflict between different groups within the health profession with very

The corporate world's influence on medical science

The influence of the corporate world on the domain of medical science has not gone unnoticed by those inside the discipline. Two recent papers on the subject describe the trend in the following manner:

Although occupational and environmental diseases are often viewed as isolated and unique failures of science, the government, or industry to protect the best interest of the public, they are in fact an outcome of a pervasive system of corporate priority setting, decision making, and influence. This system produces disease because political, economic, regulatory and ideological norms prioritize values of wealth and profit over human health and environmental well-being. Science is a key part of this system; there is a substantial tradition of manipulation of evidence, data, and analysis, ultimately designed to maintain favourable conditions for industry at both material and ideological levels. This issue offers examples of how corporations influence science, shows the effects that influence has on environmental and occupational health, and provides evidence of a systemic problem.

(Egilman and Bohme, 2005)

Corporate influences on epidemiology have become stronger and more pervasive in the last few decades, particularly in the contentious fields of pharmacoepidemiology and occupational epidemiology. For every independent epidemiologist studying the side effects of medicines and the hazardous effects of industrial chemicals, there are several other epidemiologists hired by industry to attack the research and to debunk it as "junk science." In some instances these activities have gone as far as efforts to block publication. In many instances, academics have accepted industry funding which has not been acknowledged, and only the academic affiliations of the company-funded consultants have been listed. These activities are major threats to the integrity of the field, and its survival as a scientific discipline. There is no simple solution to these problems. However, for the last two decades there has been substantial discussion on ethics in epidemiology, partly in response to the unethical conduct of many industry-funded consultants. Professional organizations, such as the International Epidemiological Association, can play a major role in encouraging and supporting epidemiologists to assert positive principles of how science should work, and how it should be applied to public policy decisions, rather than simply having a list of what not to do.

(Pearce, 2008)

Healthcare, under the influence

Can medical research be trusted? Can the scientists who sign their names to it, the journals that publish it?

These disturbing questions have been raised by a series of multi-billion-dollar lawsuits against one of the world's largest pharmaceutical firms.

Merck & Co. was forced to pull its top-selling pain medication Vioxx from the market in September of 2004, after research showed the drug increased the risk of heart attacks and strokes and may have contributed to thousands of deaths. The company agreed last year to pay $4.85-billion (U.S.) to settle the bulk of claims against it.

Internal Merck documents, filed as part of the litigation, are fuelling a debate over the role drug companies play in clinical trials —the process that underpins the testing and validation of modern medicinal treatments and new drug approvals.

Some Vioxx trials and promotional review articles were designed, executed and largely completed by drug company staff or hired hands. With the manuscript in hand, the company would then search for doctors willing to lend their reputations to the work—for a fee.

Merck denies any wrongdoing. "This is an example of trial-lawyer courtroom antics masquerading as scientific debate," said company spokesman Kent Jarrell.

Even so, Catherine DeAngelis, the outspoken editor-in-chief of *JAMA (Journal of the American Medical Association)*, said the lawsuits have opened a unique portal to view the inner workings of the drug industry. And, she said, the physicians and academics who become the guest authors of questionable studies and ghostwritten promotional articles are little more than "prostitutes."

"The profession of medicine, in every aspect—clinical, education and research —has been inundated with profound influence from the pharmaceutical and medical devices industries," Dr. DeAngelis and Phil Fontanarosa, *JAMA*'s executive deputy editor, wrote in an editorial. "This has occurred because physicians have allowed it to happen and it's time to stop."

"What she [Dr. DeAngelis] recognizes," said Arthur Schafer, director of the Centre for Professional and Applied Ethics at the University of Manitoba, "is that all of modern medicine is floating on a sea of drug company money and the result has been utterly corrosive."

Source: excerpted from Paul Taylor, "Health care, under the influence," *Globe & Mail*, April 26, 2008, p. A12.

different interests and opinions about the state of scientific research and the conditions under which that research takes place. In this conflict, corporations, especially those in the medical industry, have both the motive and the financial clout to push their particular vision successfully.

CONCLUSION

Disease is not the result of irresistible laws governed by nature, or of unhealthy lifestyle choices that are independent of socially determined political and economic factors. Medical advance did not lead the industrialized world on its incredible journey away from early death by infectious disease. The real champions, according to scholars from Szreter to Fogel, were improved living conditions through higher incomes and public safety measures. Similarly, neither the biomedical nor behavioral approach adequately explains the emergence of the major causes of death today, cancer and heart disease. Despite a massive investment of time and money on the part of the medical industry, very little progress has been made in curing cancer or even reducing the incidence of most major cancers. Heart disease mortality has shown more improvement, but again the medical community can take little credit for this change. This is not to say that genes, germs and life styles do not matter. They *do* matter, but we hope to demonstrate in Chapters 3 and 4 that, generally speaking, the environment in which germs and genes travel, and that influences individual choice, is more important in determining disease.

It follows that the primary means of reducing and effecting the character of disease is to change the working and living conditions of the population. This requires a discussion of the class nature of society and its effects on disease. In Chapters 3 and 4 we will show that the change in disease patterns in the twentieth century was a function of significant changes in the capitalist production process and therefore in the ways in which people work and live. Only by broadening our understanding of the determinants of health and disease in this way will we be able to deal effectively with health concerns in the United States.

3

TO LIVE AND DIE IN THE NINETEENTH-CENTURY UNITED STATES: A CLASS-BASED EXPLANATION OF THE RISE AND FALL OF INFECTIOUS DISEASE

Edwin Chadwick, commissioner of the Board of Health of Great Britain from 1848–1854, declared that the poorer classes in the western part of London were exposed to steady, unceasing, and sure causes of disease and death peculiar to them. "The result is the same as if twenty or thirty thousand of these people were annually taken out of their wretched dwellings and put to death" (Dubos, 1950: 130).

I have now to prove that society in England daily and hourly commits what the working-men's organs, with perfect correctness, characterize as social murder, that it has placed the workers under conditions in which they can neither retain health nor live long; that it undermines the vital force of these workers gradually, little by little, and so hurries them to the grave before their time. I have further to prove that society knows how injurious such conditions are to the health and the life of the workers, and yet does nothing to improve these conditions.

(Engels, 1850)

Economic privation proceeds by easy stages, and so long as men suffer it patiently the outside world cares little. Physical efficiency and resistance to disease slowly diminish, but life proceeds somehow, until the limit of human endurance is reached at last and counsels of despair and madness stir the sufferers from the lethargy which precedes the crisis. Then man shakes himself, and the bonds of custom are loosed. The power of ideas is sovereign, and he listens to whatever instruction of hope, illusion, or revenge is carried on the air... But who can say how much is endurable, or in what direction men will seek at last to escape from their misfortunes?

(Keynes, 1920: 250–1)

THE CASUAL HOLOCAUST

For some, the early industrial revolution in the United States was the best of times. When J. P. Morgan's daughter Louisa was married in 1900 in New York, the exclusive guest list of her closest 1,500 friends was treated to a lavish reception in the conservatory of the Morgan mansion, which had a massive extension built solely for this one-day occasion. The well-heeled guest list contributed over $1 million in gifts, including diamond jewelry, gold plates, and oriental rugs, to grace the family home of the happy couple (PBS, 1998). This chapter explores why it is that Morgan could amass such fantastic wealth, and what implications that had for the health of the broader US population.

Chapter 2 demonstrated that the decline in infectious disease in the industrial world was not driven by medical intervention. In this chapter we explain what conditions fostered infectious diseases, and what changes led to the improved living conditions and a new emphasis on public health that conquered it. The broad answer is nicely summarized by economist Anwar Shaikh. It is in the interest of business in capitalism:

> to try and push the rate of exploitation towards its social and historical limits. By the same token, it is in the interest of the subordinate classes not only to resist such efforts but also to fight against the social conditions which make this struggle necessary in the first place.
>
> (Shaikh, 1986: 167)

So the conditions for infectious disease were caused by the manner in which profits were generated in early industrial capitalism, and their amelioration was caused by the resistance and mobilization of the population to the conditions created by that particular method of generating profits.

In the mid-nineteenth century, Karl Marx argued that the greed of individual capitalists notwithstanding, the driving force of capitalism was that firms needed to continuously seek to maximize revenue and minimize cost or risk being forced out of existence by the iron discipline of competition. Marx further argued that in the formative years of capitalist development, when technological advance was not yet an established feature of the economy and hand tools were still the primary method of production, profits (which are a form of what Marx called surplus value) would come from "absolute surplus value," "produced by prolongation of the working day" (Marx, 1967 [1867]: 299).

In the absence of rapidly advancing productive technology, profits were generated by "squeezing" workers. This was possible because of an overabundance of labor caused by people being forced off the land and into cities. One example of this process was Britain's enclosure movement, which Marx so vividly described, where the privatization of communal land eliminated a crucial resource for many peasants, turning a difficult existence into one that was impossible to continue. This, coupled with the lack of effective organization of these new factory workers, made conditions ripe for low wages and poor working conditions. While most people correctly associate modern capitalism with innovations in production, early industrialization was characterized by the absolute surplus value extraction techniques of increasing the working day and holding down wages.

THE CONTEXT FOR INFECTIOUS DISEASE IN THE UNITED KINGDOM: OVERWORKED, UNDERPAID, OVERCROWDED, AND INSANITARY

Although some in the United States see their country as "exceptional," Chapter 2 showed that the United States followed the United Kingdom in terms of health transformation. This chapter will argue that the similar paths out of infectious disease in the two nations can largely be explained by the United States (and all the other second-wave industrializing nations) following the economic path first laid down by the British. This makes the British case particularly interesting and worthy of some attention as a precedent-setting, foundational example. Its role as the leader of the industrial revolution has also meant that it has been the subject of most of the scholarship and data collection on the impact of early industrial capitalism on the condition of its citizens. In very broad-brush strokes, the trail blazed by the British went from abysmal living and working conditions for most of the population to massive and successful protests that altered the structure of political and economic policy in an effort to provide a degree of protection to the typical Briton from the negative impacts of the new capitalist system.

One of the most ideologically charged debates in economic history revolves around when living standards started to improve in the United Kingdom. The optimistic view, put forward by the defenders of free market, liberal capitalism, argues that, at least after 1820 or so, incomes and living standards increased dramatically for the typical UK citizen. The pessimistic view, associated with critics of the unfettered free markets, argues that until the mid-1800s incomes were static, and that because of accompanying hardships (twelve-hour days, seven-day work weeks, and decreased access to common lands where food could be grown), living standards most likely fell. It is worth noting here that even the optimists agree that prior to 1820 incomes were stagnant. Estimating income figures from so far back in history always involves a little guesswork, but the most used figures place annual income growth per person at somewhere between 0.52 percent and 0.17 percent between 1760 and 1800. By the 1830 to 1870 period this had increased to almost 2 percent (Mokyr, 1993: 9). However, translating this into an increase in "living conditions" for the typical person is not straightforward. It is possible that the income increases were not going to workers, but went disproportionately to the capitalist class, increasing inequality. Therefore the increases in income might not mean an increase in living standards for the average citizen during the extraordinary transformation that marked early industrial capitalism in the United Kingdom.

Poverty and insecurity

> Of all of the preposterous assumptions of humanity over humanity, nothing exceeds most of the criticisms made on the habits of the poor by the well-housed, well-warmed, and well-fed.
>
> (Herman Melville)

It appears as though the pessimists are winning the day, even if living standards are narrowly defined as income. Though the British economy as a whole was growing, incomes for many in the population were stagnant or even decreasing. If income inequality is getting worse, it is possible (although not inevitable) that economic growth can be accompanied by decreased living standards for much of the population. Fogel's data suggests that this is exactly what happened. While the "lower classes" in Great Britain saw little change, or a slight decline in some regions, in their life expectancy during the nineteenth century, that of the "upper classes" increased dramatically. As a result the gap between the life expectancy of the rich and the poor increased by about ten years (Fogel, 2004: 36). At around 1815, a fully grown male from the upper classes was five inches taller than a male worker (Fogel, 2004: 40). The average height (a proxy for nutrition) of British workers was lower in 1850 than it was in the earlier years of the century (Mokyr, 1993: 127). Economic growth may be a necessary condition for increasing living standards over time, but is not sufficient, in and of itself, to ensure that the average person in society will enjoy income gains. The health gradient also provides evidence for the hypothesis that profits were driven, to a large extent, by methods that squeezed workers by holding down wages, for work of long hours in unhealthy conditions.

If the average resident of the United Kingdom enjoyed income gains, this should be reflected in an increase in consumption. However, there seems to be little evidence of working-class consumption increase, and considerable evidence to the contrary (Mokyr, 1993: 127–8). Between 1800 and 1850 the population of London doubled, but the number of cattle and sheep slaughtered only increased by 46 percent and 76 percent respectively. The consumption of milk per person during this period fell, as did the amount of wheat available per capita (Hobsbawm, 1964: 84–7). Fogel argued that the reason that life expectancy increased so little in the United Kingdom prior to 1890 was the limited quality and quantity of food that was consumed by the "ordinary" English family (Fogel, 2004: 9).

Even if the optimists are correct, and incomes of the average UK resident did begin to rise in 1820 rather than 1850, there is absolutely no doubt that income tended to remain close to, or occasionally fell below, levels of real biological subsistence for many members of the work force until the last half of the 1800s. As late as the 1840s, 10 percent of the population were paupers— the permanent, hard-core poor (Hobsbawm, 1964: 73). Existence was so marginal that spells of unemployment, a common feature of the economically unstable landscape, would inevitably result in catastrophe. For example, during the economic downturn of 1826 in Lancashire somewhere between 30 and 70 percent of the population was completely destitute (Hobsbawm, 1964: 75).

Even in good times, wages were precarious at best. In a good year, 1851, in Preston, 52 percent of all working-class families with

Public policy: the Poor Law Amendment Act of 1834

It was not only the enclosure movement that created a large and desperate workforce in early nineteenth-century England. The much-reviled Poor Law Amendment (or New Poor Law) passed in 1834 was expressly designed to force laborers into the workforce by making public assistance as miserly and miserable as possible.

Prior to the 1834 Amendment, the amount that the government was spending supporting the poor was increasing. Relief spending in England increased from 1 percent of GDP in 1750 to 2 percent in 1831 (Boyer, 2010). Not only was this considered to be a drain on the taxpaying middle and upper classes, it also allowed the common laborer to forsake a life of honest and morally valuable work to take up a life of indolence and sloth—a condition called "pauperism." Unemployment was not seen as a problem of insufficient demand for labor, but a consequence of the personal deficiencies of the worker. As Lynn Lees wrote: "To the question, what ought the state do for the poor? They answered, 'less'" (1998: 116).

The New Poor Laws stipulated an end to "outdoor" relief, which meant that the only way in which an "able-bodied" man could claim assistance was to enter the "indoor" relief of the workhouse. According to the New Poor Laws, the public workhouse needed to be so abhorrent that it made even the most grueling of wage labor a superior alternative. Paupers entering the workhouse underwent a degrading initiation in which they gave up their clothes in exchange for an "ill-fitting uniform" and severe haircut. All personal possessions were confiscated. The nine or ten-hour workday started at 5 am in the summer and 7 am in the winter. The entire day was strictly accounted for by working, eating, sleeping, and religious services, under the belief that thorough regimentation would cure the paupers of their lack of discipline (Lees, 1998: 147). In regions where workhouses had not yet been constructed, or where there were too many poor to squeeze into already overcrowded indoor relief, outdoor relief was still offered but only under the overarching condition that, like the workhouse, it must be as wretched as possible. Assistance could only be offered at levels that were less than the local wage. In exchange for their meager government assistance, recipients were put to work doing particularly nasty jobs such as breaking stones or grinding corn by hand (Lees, 1998: 146).

According to Lees, "the residualist welfare state of earlier times was renegotiated into a far harsher form by a middle- and upper-class public determined to combat the 'pauperization' of the social body, at the same time as they defended their pocketbooks" (Lees, 1998: 116). The desperate workforce created by the New Poor Laws also had the very predictable, and intended, effect of depressing wages in early industrializing Britain.

children below working age, employed full time in a solid trade, did not earn enough to rise above the poverty line (Hobsbawm, 1975: 221). This was also not a problem isolated to a few unfortunate cities. Rural wages were actually considerably lower. In the late 1700s the wages of unskilled laborers were so low that they would have "sunk below the starvation level" were it not for miserly and punitive programs of government assistance (Polanyi, 1944: 93).

Another bit of evidence on the paucity of working-class purchasing power is the substandard goods they were forced to purchase. In a *Lancet* enquiry during the 1850s all of the bread, all the butter, half of the oatmeal, and just under half of the milk was adulterated (Hobsbawm, 1964: 84–7). The poor could only very rarely afford woolen clothing, mostly wearing patches purchased at the local pawnbroker, to protect them from England's notoriously cold and damp climate (Engels, 1850: 66–7). The low level of wages made it necessary for all "exchangeable" members of the worker's family to sell their labor power in the market. The expansion of plant size, mechanization of trade, and dilution of skills dramatically increased the proportion of women and children in the fledgling industrial sector. Prior to 1850, there is no question that the standard of living of the vast majority of society was a constant struggle against absolute poverty.

Environmental conditions

If a broader definition of living standards is used, which includes living and working conditions, the pessimistic case becomes even stronger. Early industrial capitalism was marked by a growing concentration of manufacturing in large cities, because the demands of competition required cost-minimizing capitalists to be near large numbers of workers, transportation, and raw materials. Cities, increasingly crowded with low-waged workers who lacked the political power to improve public health, resulted in housing and sanitary conditions that made infectious disease epidemics the

Friedrich Engels on *The Conditions of the Working Class*

The workers get what is too bad for the property holding class. In the great towns of England everything may be had of the best, but it costs money and the workman, who must keep house on a couple of pence, cannot afford much expense .... The potatoes which the workers buy are usually poor, the vegetables wilted, the cheese old and of poor quality, the bacon rancid, the meat lean, tough, taken from old, often diseased, cattle, or such as have died a natural death, and not fresh even then, often half decayed. ... The meat, which the workers buy, is very often past using; but having bought it, they must eat it.

(Engels, 1850: 68)

The quantity of food varies, of course, like its quality, according to the rate of wages, so that among ill-paid workers, even if they have no large families, hunger prevails in spite of full and regular work; and the number of the ill paid is very large. Especially in London, where the competition of the workers rises with the increase of population, this class is very numerous, but it is to be found in other towns as well. In these cases all sorts of devices are used; potato parings, vegetable refuse, and rotten vegetables are eaten for want of other food, and everything greedily gathered up which may possibly contain an atom of nourishment. And, if the week's wages are used up before the end of the week, it often happens that in the closing days the family gets only as much food if any, as is barely sufficient to keep off starvation. Of course, such a way of living unavoidably engenders a multitude of diseases, and when these appear, when the father from whose work the family is chiefly supported, whose physical exertion most demands nourishment, and who therefore first succumbs—when the father is utterly disabled, then misery reaches its heights, and then the brutality with which society abandons its members, just when their need is greatest, comes out fully into the light of day.

(Engels, 1850: 73)

typical conditions. Evidence suggests that the lack of improvement in mortality between 1820 and 1870 was in large part because of the greater spread of disease in newly enlarged cities. In the "little Ireland" section of Manchester there was one toilet for every 125 people (Rosen, 1958: 205). In the 1840s, London sewage was pumped directly into the River Thames, creating an unpleasant lingering odor as well as creating waterborne health hazards (McKeown, 1976b: 125). Housing was a particular problem. The influx of people into the cities resulted in a sharp increase in the price of rental housing. Cash-strapped urban families responded by crowding into increasingly tiny dwellings which were stacked ever closer together (Williamson, 1994: 350). Builders attempting to make a profit on expensive land increasingly took short cuts with materials and standards. Even staunch free market economist Nassau Senior had this to say on the condition of the great British towns:

> What other result can be expected when any man can purchase or hire a plot of ground, is allowed to cover it with such buildings as he may think fit, where there is not power to enforce drainage or sewerage, or to regulate the width of the streets, or to prevent houses from being packed back to back ... or their being filled with as many inmates as their walls can contain.
>
> (cited in Flinn, 1965: 39)

Landlords must "be compelled by law, though it should cost them a percentage of their rent and profit, to take measures which shall prevent the towns which they create from being the centers of disease" (Flinn, 1965: 39).

The effect of insanitary conditions was larger, and the spread of disease was easier, in bigger, more crowded cities (Cutler et al., 2006: 102). As a result, the death rates and infant mortality in cities were considerably higher than those in rural areas (Williamson, 1994: 335, 352). Mortality rates also rose sharply in the large British cities between 1831 and 1841 (see Table 3.1). Karl Polanyi memorably summarized the condition of the urban worker: "Dumped into this

Table 3.1 Mortality rate per 1,000 of population, selected major UK industrial cities

	1831	1844
Birmingham	14.6	27.2
Bristol	16.9	31.0
Liverpool	21.0	34.8
Manchester	30.2	33.8

Source: Rosen (1958: 202).

bleak slough of misery, the immigrant peasant, or even the former yeoman or copyholder was soon transformed into a nondescript animal of the mire" (1944: 99).

In addition to these broad social killers, specific occupations carried their own unique hazards. In Sheffield, knife grinders suffered in increasing numbers from "grinders' disease" (silicosis) in the 1800s precisely because more workers were packed into smaller shops, which were in turn packed into a bigger, dirtier city (Hobsbawm, 1964: 117). "A black pigmentation of the lung," or black lung, was a common cause of death among coal miners. Chimney sweeps had a greater incidence of skin cancer. Lung cancer was rife in metal miners (Seaton, 2000: 1404). Since these illnesses, and many other occupational diseases, were confined to specific jobs, no single one of them spread widely enough to constitute an epidemic as did the infectious diseases that were the mass killers, but taken collectively they constituted yet another source of suffering for the already vulnerable workers during the industrial revolution.

In 1866, Florence Nightingale refused a request to open a new children's hospital. Her explanation was that opening more hospitals was not a remedy for infant mortality and sickness, which could only be solved by improving conditions in the children's environment (Brierley, 1970: 98). Early industrial capitalism, dominated by absolute surplus value techniques, resulted in workers and their families being underfed, improperly sheltered, poorly clothed, and overworked, inhibiting their immune system from working, effectively creating an "epidemic constitution" for infectious disease (Chernomas, 1999; Chernomas and Hudson, 2007; Dubos, 1959, 1965; Galdston, 1954).

Marginal productivity theory

The welfare of the laboring classes depends on whether they get much or little; but their attitude toward the other classes—and, therefore, the stability of the social state depends chiefly on the question, whether the amount that they get, be it large or small, is what they produce. If they create a small amount of wealth and get the whole of it, they may not seek to revolutionize society; but if it were to appear that they produce an ample amount and get only a part of it, many of them would become revolutionists, and all would have the right to do so.

(John Bates Clark, 1899: 4)

The explanation of the improvements in living conditions of the working class in this book is dramatically different from that of many economists. The standard explanation for how incomes are determined, both over time and within a society at any moment in time, is called marginal productivity theory. The more colloquial version of this theory is that people "get what they deserve," or "earn what they are worth." In the language of mainstream economics, people are paid their marginal revenue product, which is equal to the value of their productivity. The more an individual can produce and the higher the value that this production can be sold for, the higher the income. This theory explains income distribution at any moment in time between members of society by suggesting that those who do things that are valuable to society, like produce more, or produce things of higher value, will be paid more. Thus, Clark, the US neoclassical economist, believes that workers receive what they produce. This theory also purports to explain income growth over time. People are richer now than they were in the past because their productivity has increased. Thanks to diligent capitalists, spurred by the competitive drive, improved technology means that every worker today produces a great deal more than workers in the past. Similarly, as workers improve their ability to produce through improved literacy and better education, their incomes, and society's collective wealth, will rise.

But people are often not paid their marginal productivity. As Nobel Prize winning economist Joseph Stiglitz recently argued, the theory was originally intended to "justify the vast inequalities that seemed so troubling in the mid-19th century." He continues:

It is a theory that has always been cherished by the rich. Evidence for its validity, however, remains thin. The corporate executives who helped bring on the recession of the past three years—whose contribution to our society, and to their own companies, has been massively negative—went on to receive large bonuses. In some cases, companies were so embarrassed about calling such rewards "performance bonuses" that they felt compelled to change the name to "retention bonuses" (even if the only thing being retained was bad performance). Those who have contributed great positive innovations to our society, from the pioneers of genetic understanding to the pioneers of the Information Age, have received a pittance compared with those responsible for the financial innovations that brought our global economy to the brink of ruin.

(Stiglitz, 2011)

The second connection between productivity and rising incomes over time is, of course, in part true. The total value of goods and services produced in our economy is far greater now that it was at the dawn of the twentieth century. By definition, this means that average incomes must be rising. However, in contrast to marginal productivity theory, this book argues that while increased productivity is necessary for increased incomes, on its own it may not be sufficient to improve the lot of the "average" citizen. How income is distributed will depend more on the ability of groups in society to capture productivity gains. For example, we will show in Chapters 3 and 4 that in the late nineteenth and late twentieth centuries, productivity gains have gone disproportionately to the wealthier members of society. In both periods this was the result of policies and economic conditions that favored employers at the expense of employees. To take the latter example, Figure 3.1 shows the trends in productivity growth and wages in the United States from 1960 to 2000. Between 1960 and 1975, the wages trend went upwards in parallel with productivity. In fact, for a time, wages grew slightly more quickly than productivity. However, starting around 1980 a dramatic change occurred in the US economy. Wages stagnated while productivity grew. We will delve

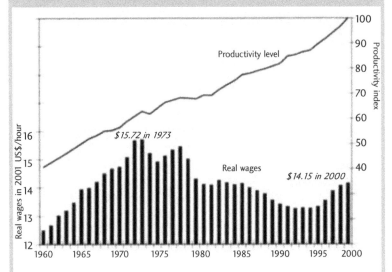

Figure 3.1 Average real wages and productivity levels in the United States, 1960 to 2000 (average earnings in 2001 dollars, nonsupervisory private sector)

Source: Pollin (2003: 43).

into the explanation for this in Chapter 4, but for now it suffices to demonstrate that there is no magic, inevitable connection between productivity and wages. The working population can earn more only with a combination of productivity gains and a successful struggle to wrest a portion of the income generated by that productivity from firms.

THE UK TRANSITION

If the principal cause of infectious disease was the abysmal conditions in which people lived, the triumph over these illnesses came from an end to these conditions. In the last quarter of the nineteenth century, workers' struggles for better working and living conditions and increased wages grew in militancy and effectiveness. An increasing number of strikes, many of which featured violent confrontations between business and workers, led to the formation of militant unions, left-wing political parties, and to the advancement of a social reform agenda that included rising wages, the legislation of a shorter work day, and regulation that placed restrictions on the employment of women, children, and the conditions of work. The result was improved nutrition, housing, and clothing.

In the most advanced industrialized capitalist country of the time, the United Kingdom, this happened earlier than in other nations. In *The Great Transformation*, Polanyi (1944) argued that the literally deadly consequences of leaving income and living conditions to the free market in the early years of the industrial revolution resulted in a protective countermovement in the last half of the 1800s.

The British Factory Act of 1833 indicated the abysmal labor conditions of the time and was an early precursor of the protective movement that would gather force in later decades. According to the provisions of the Act, children under 9 years old had to go to school, those between 9 and 13 years old had their work day limited to eight hours a day, and teenagers between 14 and 18 years old could work no more than twelve hours a day. The Act also prohibited cleaning machinery while it was in motion, a practice that was cost-effective because it reduced capital downtime, but had obvious risks for the unfortunate cleaner.

Polanyi argues that after 1850, the nascent working class and the fading aristocracy combined to sweep in transformative rules that would protect society from the ruination of the market (Polanyi,

1944: 155). The list of interventions is long, but crucially included extending the Mines Act to prohibit hiring boys under 12 years old "not attending schools and unable to read or write," making single-shaft coal mines illegal, and legalizing mine inspections (Polanyi, 1944: 146). Over time the Factory Acts were strengthened to include the ten-hour day for women and children in textiles in 1847 and the rest of industry in 1867, which placed an important limit on the ability of firms to earn profits by simply having employees toil in ever-longer shifts. It is this change that, one economist argued, caused, "the zeal for technology" among British owners.

The newly legal trade union movement made bargaining over the spoils from the newly installed technology one of its specific objectives (Von Tunzelmann, 1994: 296). Perhaps the most important change was making trade unions and strikes legal in 1875 (Hobsbawm, 1975: 27). It is worth noting that every one of these legislative changes, from reduced hours to increased safety in the mines, was opposed with great determination, something that reflected "little credit on the coal owners, the manufacturers and their spokesmen" (Rosen, 1958: 268).

As a result of these changes to both worker incomes and the environments in which they worked and lived, living standards improved markedly in the last half of the nineteenth century. Fruit became a part of the average diet for the British people after 1870. What was true for food became true for working-class consumption in general. Rising incomes led to factory production for a specific working-class market for the first time. Clothing and shoe stores, for example, began to multiply. By 1875 there were already 300 shoe stores in the United Kingdom; by 1900 there were 2,600 (Hobsbawm, 1974: 160–3).

Some improvements were also made to the abysmal condition of British cities. One of the first champions of public health, Edwin Chadwick, worked tirelessly to decrease the incidence of illness among the poor by improving their living environment. Correctly speculating that it would be easier to transform the outside environment than it would be to increase the standard of living of the poor, Chadwick agued for a sweeping municipal cleanliness program, including drainage, street cleaning, water supplies, sewers, and removal of noxious refuse (Rosen, 1958: 215). His example spawned civic reform groups across the United Kingdom prior to 1850, worried that the continued misery of the working population might lead to proletarian upheaval (Rosen, 1958: 219).

Yet these movements had no real impact on policy until the

1848 cholera epidemic in Liverpool scared the government into creating its first General Board of Health. It met with such strong opposition that it only lasted five years (until 1854). It was criticized on philosophical grounds for compromising private property rights and reducing freedom when it encouraged towns to impose taxes to finance sanitary facilities (Szreter, 2003: 422; Porter, 1999: 120). An article criticizing the Board in *The Times* argued that "we prefer to take our chance of cholera and the rest than be bullied into health" (Rosen, 1958: 200). It was also opposed by the vested interests that were harmed by its actions. For example, water companies were threatened by proposals to deliver a safe municipal water supply. Despite the short tenure of the Board, some real improvements were made. It was during this period that sewer systems and water supplies were built in larger communities.

The large expansion of public health infrastructure would have to wait until later in the century, after the vote was expanded, due to pressure by at first the male working class, then female citizens. These new voters changed political realities, especially at the local level (Szreter, 2004a: 83). After much delay and constant pressure from both the new urban workers and the middle-class reform movement, towns began the construction of sewers and home water connections around 1870 (Szreter, 2004b: 707). An 1879 survey found that most large urban communities had adequate supplies of water in terms of quantity, even if the quality was not always quite what might have been hoped for (Rosen, 1958: 232). There was also legislation targeted more specifically to benefit the poorer working populations. Zoning and housing regulations accompanied food inspections to ensure that workers were at least getting the food they paid for, which as we have seen was often not the case (Baldwin, 1999: 539; Polanyi, 1944: 146). In 1860 the government started inspecting food and drink (Polanyi, 1944: 146). By 1905 local governments in the United Kingdom had embarked on a massive campaign of spending on health and environmental measures (Szreter, 2004a: 83).

During the first decades of the industrial revolution, wages and working conditions could only be described at best as marginally adequate to sustain life. The standards of nutrition, protection from the elements, sleep and rest time, sanitary conditions, child labor and labor in general corresponded to those of the poorest countries of the contemporary world, with mortality and morbidity rates to match. In those areas where most people had insufficient nutrition, sanitation, clothing, and housing, the major causes of death were tuberculosis, pneumonia, measles, diarrhea, and other infectious diseases. All of the diseases that dominated nineteenth-century society's mortality statistics began to recede only with the change in social and economic conditions as working-class consumption, sanitation, working hours, and labor conditions improved. This shift in the pattern of disease began prior to the discovery of the germ "responsible" or the medical antidote invented.

Every once in a while copying the British is a good idea. Just as the UK population escaped from early death by infectious disease through a combination of increased incomes and public health measures, so too did every other industrial nation. In this the United States was no exception. The US experience differed from that of Britain in some important ways. US industrialization began later. As we will show in this section, its shock was not quite as devastating, and the Progressive period, which was the US equivalent of the late nineteenth-century reforms, relied less heavily on government solutions. Yet the story of the US emergence from early death and infectious disease in many ways mirrors the example set by the United Kingdom.

Recall Figure 2.2 from Chapter 2. According to Fogel's data on life expectancy, in 1800 people in the United States fared considerably better than those in the United Kingdom on average. Yet by 1900 life expectancy in the United States had not improved at all. In fact, life expectancy was lower in 1900 than it was in 1800. It is only after 1900 that life expectancy in the United States started to improve dramatically. Just as was the case in the United Kingdom during this economic period, the major causes of death in the United States were from infectious disease.

The fact that life expectancy in the United States only really improved after 1900 should not come as a surprise since, in broad strokes, the picture of the US past looks like a great deal like that of the United Kingdom. The early stages of the US industrial revolution were marked by the problems associated with generating profits by "squeezing" workers with longer hours and lower wages, in a political environment in which government would very reliably (and sometimes violently) side with business in any dispute with labor. The results of this early stage of industrialization were traumatic enough to generate widespread, often fierce protest. Only with the success of these protests and the introduction of the famed Progressive period did the living conditions for many in the United States improve sufficiently to escape the trap of infectious disease.

THE CONTEXT FOR INFECTIOUS DISEASE IN THE
UNITED STATES: OVERWORKED, UNDERPAID,
OVERCROWDED, AND INSANITARY

In the United Kingdom the pessimists have made a strong case that living standards actually fell before 1850. The United States, in contrast, does not seem to have suffered such a traumatic transformation to early industrial capitalism. Real GDP per capita in the United States grew at an average annual rate of 1.3 percent, resulting in an increase in income per person from $1,200 in 1820 to $2,445 in 1870 (Maddison, 2001: tables A-1c and A-1d), and some of the increase even made its way to some members of the working class. Between 1850 and 1890 real wages increased by around 50 percent, although it needs to be remembered that this modest increase started from low levels and was still not sufficient to move many workers out of outright poverty (Dubofsky, 1996: 18). Of course, rising real wages only increase family incomes if a person is actually employed, which was far from guaranteed during this period. There are the further questions of how these incomes were distributed and whether the deterioration of living and working conditions during this period overwhelmed any income gains. A small increase in wages along with a 70-hour work week in a dangerous and insanitary mine or factory without access to land where food can be grown is not a prescription for improved health indicators.

Moreover, the economic benefits in the late nineteenth century were going disproportionately to the very richest US citizens. While data during this period is difficult to come by, the information available suggests that the period was one of rising inequality (Rosenbloom and Stutes, 2008: 147). In 1916, the top 1 percent of the population owned 40 percent of the total wealth in the United States. This marked a substantial increase from the 1870 Census (which, though based on self-reported wealth, was not, the authors claimed, systematically biased in any way), in which the wealthiest 1 percent owned a lower, although still impressive, 28 percent of total property in the nation. That the same figure stood at 22.5 percent in 1949, after the equalizing effects of the Second World War and at the beginning of the golden age of growth, is telling. The idea that the economic development in the United States was benefiting those at very upper echelons of the income spectrum well into the twentieth century is strengthened by the fact that the degree of wealth inequality was much higher in the more industrialized states of Connecticut, where the top 1 percent owned 41 percent of the property, and Massachusetts, where they owned 35 percent, than was the case in the more agricultural states (at least all of those that did not have a legacy of slavery) (Rosenbloom and Stutes, 2008: 150). To further reinforce this point, US workers, who comprised the majority of the population in urban areas, owned at most 5 percent of urban wealth (Pessen, 1976).

It is not just that such inequality is bad for health outcomes, although this is certainly true. It is also about income between different classes of people in society. The top 1 percent was made up primarily of owners, who were receiving a larger and larger share of the national income during this period. Part of what was generating this was an economic system that relied heavily on the impoverishment of much of the rest of the population. This did not only create inequality, it also kept people in poverty and working in dangerous conditions longer than would have been the case if the benefits of economic growth were more evenly shared.

Poverty and insecurity

In the United States, a small portion of workers fared quite well. Labor historian Melvyn Dubofsky argued that during the 1870s and 1880s the aristocrats of US labor were responsible for organizing work, deciding its pace, and even determining how pay would be distributed among the workers (Dubofsky, 1996: 37). The top 15 percent of workers, who possessed specific skills and technical ability, could earn as much as $800 to $1,100 a year, enough to afford a respectable middle-class lifestyle. These jobs, which included trades like iron rollers, locomotive engineers, pattern makers, and glass blowers, were jobs that required considerable responsibility and experience (Montgomery, 1976).

On the other hand in the late nineteenth century, few would have envied the position of the unskilled worker in the fledgling US industrial sector. While wages were certainly growing for the average person, they were still dangerously low and precariously unstable for many workers. Wages, especially of unskilled labor, were kept in check by inflows of workers from two sources. People streamed off farms as agricultural production became increasingly capital intensive. They also arrived from other countries in growing numbers. In 1870, about one-third of the manufacturing work force was foreign born. Between 1865 and 1900 an amazing 12 million foreigners crossed the ocean to live in the United States (Montgomery, 1976). Immigrants, largely unskilled, with few savings or social networks, and often excluded by both trade and ethnicity from the unions that did exist, would often work at wages well below their domestic counterparts. At the Homestead plant (to which we will return) in 1907 weekly wages for a white worker were $22, for Irish and Scots $16, and for "Slavs" a risible $12 (Heilbroner, 1977: 129).

Of course, the waves of immigrants also increased the supply of unskilled labor, putting downward pressure on wage rates in general. In 1880, about 45 percent of workers could, if they remained lucky enough to avoid the twin working-class disasters of illness or accident, just afford the basic necessities. A further 40 percent of working families could not afford even a basic basket of necessities, and about one-quarter of these lived in absolute penury (Montgomery, 1976). By the early 1900s, over $800 per annum was needed to sustain a typical working-class family of four in New York. Yet a survey by the US Commission on Immigration found an average yearly income for a male worker of $413, with almost half of the 10,000 workers sampled earning below $400. Female workers earned about half as much as men (Dubofsky, 1996: 22).

It is no wonder that younger family members were forced to work to supplement the family income. In the 1830s in New England somewhere between one-third and half of the entire labor force was under 16 years old (Pessen, 1976). In the coalmines, one union representative claimed that it was necessary for the father "to take the child into the mine with him to assist in winning bread for the family" (Heilbroner, 1977: 133). Even as late as 1900 there were at least 1.7 million children engaged in paid labor in the United States (Rosen, 1958: 428). A reporter describing the children in the mill towns around Pittsburgh wrote, "their eyes gleam with premature knowledge, which is the result of daily struggle, not for life, but for existence" (Dubofsky, 1996: 22).

Even after conditions started to improve in the early 1900s, working lives could best be described as perilous. Studies at the time by the US Children's Bureau showed that low incomes had an important impact on children's health. A study in 1915 found that families where the father had an annual income of less than $450 had an infant death rate of 157 in every 1,000 births. If the father's income was $1,850 the mortality rate was less than a quarter of that—only 37 in 1,000 (Fitch, 1924: 58). Given the poor living and working conditions, illness was common. With the lack of support for the non-working, illness for the head of the family was also devastating. In the three months of a 1917–18 study by the New York City Department of Health, illness struck each family once on average. Hardship as a result of illness was so great that families were forced to dramatically reduce spending on food. Thirty-nine percent of families removed meat, 40 percent cut out eggs, and 14 percent eliminated milk from children's diets. Given the connection between living conditions and health stressed in this book, it should be no surprise that the report concluded that in 13 percent of the cases recovery was definitely slowed by poor living standards (Fitch, 1924: 58).

The other great threat to the workers' livelihood was unemployment. This was a particular threat in the later stages of the nineteenth century, which experienced a series of serious economic downturns. For example, workers in the anthracite coalmines of Pennsylvania managed only an average of 178 days of work a year during the prolonged downturn between 1893 and 1898 (Montgomery, 1976). Periods of joblessness were a common feature of even good times because of the seasonal and temporary nature of much work. With no state relief and private charities glaringly insufficient and often demeaning, unemployment often resulted in at least temporary destitution.

An 1885 study found that one-third of the immigrant workforce and one-quarter of those born in the United States had a substantial bout of unemployment every year. The native-born numbers actually represent an understatement of the insecurity facing the blue-collar workforce, since they include much more stable white-collar employment. Bouts of unemployment for the blue-collar US born workforce were virtually identical to those of the immigrant population (Keyssar, 1986: 80). High unemployment rates also hurt those fortunate enough to retain their jobs, since excess labor forces down wages. During the recessionary decade of the 1870s in New York, the daily wage for an artisan in the building industry dropped from $2.50–$3.00 for eight hours in 1872 to $1.50–$2.00 for ten hours in 1875 (Heilbroner, 1977: 133). As Heilbroner observed, "When a man enjoys an increase in pay for, say, nine years, but is unemployed for the tenth, it is hard to say that his standard of living has risen" (1977: 133).

Essentially, many US workers were paid so little that they were very susceptible to infectious disease. As we shall see, this was not an inevitable consequence of a particular stage of US development, but a result of a very deliberate set of conditions that favored capital over labor.

Conditions of work

These miserly incomes were despite a working week that could only be described as crushing. According to a report published in 1893 for the Senate Committee of Finance (called the Aldrich Report after chair Nelson Aldrich), average weekly hours in manufacturing in 1850 were a backbreaking 69 hours (see Figure 3.2). This declined slowly but steadily at an average of 0.225 hours per year over the next 40 years, so that by 1890 the working week stood at a still lengthy 60 hours. According to the Census of Manufacturers, which started in 1900, the weekly work burden dropped by a more rapid 0.32 per year to 55.5 hours by 1914 (Whaples, 2010). Remember that these are average hours, so some unfortunate souls toiled for considerably longer.

In the steel industry in the United States during this period, men worked twelve hours a day, seven days a week. Transit workers labored seven days a week, 14 hours a day. It was not uncommon for girls working in the laundry industry to work 16, 18, or even 20 hours a day amidst poor ventilation, heat and dampness (Foner, 1947 vol. 3: 12–20). At the legendary Homestead mill owned by Andrew Carnegie, workers put in a twelve-hour day every single day of the year except Christmas and, in a nod to patriotism, July 4. The only alteration of this routine was a swing shift every other week, where employees worked 24 hours straight (Heilbroner, 1977: 126). The daily grind was so onerous on working people at this time

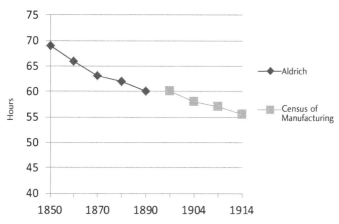

Figure 3.2 Weekly hours of work in US manufacturing

Source: Whaples (2001).

that it was often the major workplace grievance and cause of strike action. It was a factor in 25 percent of strikes, second only to wages in terms of causes, between 1881 and 1906 (Fitch, 1924: 12).

It was not only long hours that were a problem for the fledgling US workforce. The conditions in which those hours were spent were also very damaging. Returning again to Carnegie's Homestead mill, there were no lunch periods or showers and only very rudimentary sanitary facilities. Novelist Hamlin Garland's account of the factory was of "pits gaping like the mouth of hell and ovens emitting a terrible degree of heat, with grimy men filling and lining them. One man jumps down, works desperately for a few minutes and is then pulled up, exhausted. Another immediately takes his place" (cited in Heilbroner, 1977: 128). Another account claimed that because of the "maddening screech of cold saws ripping through steel," workers almost inevitably became hard of hearing. By the end of the day they were covered with "shiny grains of steel." Unsurprisingly, workers complained frequently of respiratory ailments (Wolff, 1965: 37).

These kind of dangerous conditions resulted in a predictably grisly rate of accidents and injuries. In 1893 alone in Homestead there were seven fatalities and two injuries requiring amputation. In the iron and steel mills of Pittsburgh 195 workers were killed in one year (Heilbroner, 1977: 128). In the year of 1906–07 in Pittsburgh 526 workers were killed in job accidents. In coal mining, the annual death toll never dropped below 2,000 between 1905 and 1920. On the railroad, one out of every 26 workers were injured and one in 400 killed in 1901 (Dubofsky, 1996: 24). Between 1888 and 1908 an estimated 35,000 workers were killed and 536,000 injured on average each year (Weinstein, 1968: 40). To make matters worse, compensation for these deaths and injuries was simply not considered at the time. Not only were there no public or employer insurance schemes, litigation was also unlikely to produce any favorable results for the injured party. In one famous case, a woman lost her arm in the gears of an unprotected grinding machine. State laws stipulated that the gears should be covered. The victim had complained about the exposed gears to her employer, who told her she could either accept the conditions or quit. The judge ruled that she was not eligible for damages because she had known of the risks and implicitly accepted them by not quitting (Weinstein, 1968: 42).

The conditions of work negatively impacted worker health and longevity in three ways. Most obviously, industrial accidents could result in early death or injury. Second, hazards like particulate matter in the air could lead to longer-term health problems. Finally, long hours of physically exhausting labor without sufficient recuperative time can weaken workers' ability to resist disease. All of these problems were the result of the system of industrial production in which employers steadfastly refused to incur the additional costs of providing a healthier work environment.

Environmental conditions

As was the case in the United Kingdom, low incomes and rapid urbanization meant that people's out-of-work lives were as dangerous as their place of work. The town of Homestead was scarcely more appealing that the mill. According to Garland, "The streets of the town were horrible; the building poor; the sidewalks were waylaying, sunken and full of holes .... Everywhere the yellow muck of the street lay kneaded into a sticky mass, through which groups of pale lean men slouched in faded garments, grimy with soot and grease of the mills" (cited in Heilbroner, 1977: 126). New York's Tenth Ward was said to be the most crowded district in the world; provisions for sanitation were non-existent and "cubby-hole" sized rooms doubled as workshops (Foner, 1947 vol. 2: 23).

In New York City, the population living in tenements more than tripled, from 468,000 in 1869 to 1.5 million in 1900. As many as twelve families (not individuals) would often live on one floor. Conditions were sufficiently deplorable that the legislature felt compelled to pass an act that ensured that residential buildings contained one toilet for every 21 inhabitants (although it could be located in the back yard), roofs in proper repair, and proper ventilation (Heilbroner, 1977: 152). According to an investigation of Chicago tenements in 1883–4, the streets were filled with decaying matter and filth. The housing where thousands of people lived violated all rules for drainage, plumbing, light, ventilation, and safety (Foner, 1947 vol. 2: 23). A middle-class observer described a working-class neighborhood in the following manner: "filth everywhere, trampled into sidewalks, lying in windows, collected in the eddies of doorsteps." While we might discount this as a coddled well-to-do observer's shock at how the other half lives, a recent immigrant and resident of one such neighborhood argued that his new life in the United States was "the freedom for respectable citizens to sell cabbages from hideous carts, the opportunity to live in those monstrous, dirty caves that shut out the sunshine" (cited in Heilbroner, 1977: 28). The link between the dismal living conditions of so many and infectious disease was no secret at the time. An 1858 report on health in New York City linked the high mortality to tenement housing, poor light, bad ventilation, filthy streets, and insufficient sewers (Brieger, 1997: 438). Yet repeated pleas by for sanitary reform fell on deaf ears for decades.

Employers and the state confront unions over the social determinants of health

So at the turn of the twentieth century the United States looked a lot like Britain in the 1850s. While it is true that, on average, incomes were growing in the United States faster than in Britain, and that wages for the working population at this early stage of industrialism were above those in the United Kingdom at a similar stage of development, this would have been little comfort to the millions of people living in poverty, perpetually terrified about whether they would be employed next month, working long hours in dangerous conditions for the privilege of putting a very leaky roof over their heads in a filthy and overcrowded tenement. These were the conditions that created an epidemic of infectious disease. Needless to say, the working population was not enamored of these conditions. The late 1800s and early 1900s witnessed cascading labor unrest in the United States, in both frequency and animosity, as the workers attempted to wrest a larger share of the national income away from owners. Yet low wages, long hours, and hazardous conditions remained because these conditions created profits for owners in this early stage of industrial capitalism. In their steadfast opposition to cost-increasing improvements to the life of US workers, owners could count on the support of the government.

The strike at Homestead (see box opposite) offers a glimpse into a level of violence and conflict that is no longer a part of the labor relations landscape in the United States, but was par for the course at the time. Strikes were remarkably common and commonly violent. Between 1881 and 1890 the Bureau of Labor Statistics registered 9,668 strikes or lockouts (Dubofsky, 1996: 39–40). They also featured a level of hostility that would be unheard of in today's more bureaucratic labor relations. In its outlines, the Homestead conflict was similar to countless others from Haymarket in Chicago to Bay View, Wisconsin. Despite this unrest, with the aid of the government, owners were generally able to resist even the most basic of workers' demands. It must be remembered that these were the days when firms were not required by law to negotiate with unions. Many owners were adamantly opposed to any collective action by their employees, seeing it as an imposition on employers' unilateral decision-making power in the firm. John Fitch recounted that at one of the "largest manufacturing establishments" in the country, a group of workers presented the superintendent with a petition requesting a wage increase. The superintendent not only refused to accept the petition, but also insisted that all of the signatories erase their names. The men who were either brave or stubborn enough to refuse were immediately let go (Fitch, 1924: 162).

A wide variety of strong-arm tactics were employed to tame the

Homestead

One particularly dramatic example of labor conflict occurred at the Homestead mill in July 1892. It has become famous in US labor history because of the degree of violence, the fame of Andrew Carnegie, and the strength of the Amalgamated Association of Iron and Steel Workers, which had managed to protect its workers from the ravages of the 1880s that had affected other workers in Pennsylvania. The immediate flashpoint for the lockout was that during difficult economic times, management demanded an 18 percent wage reduction, which workers were understandably reluctant to agree to.

In response to the union's recalcitrant attitude, the chief of Homestead operations, Henry Frick, locked out the workers, with plans to operate with an entirely new workforce. In an effort to prevent this, a couple of days later workers seized the mill and effectively blockaded the town. Five days later 300 men of the famous union-busting Pinkerton Agency attempted to retake the mill, and became embroiled in a vicious fight that left three Pinkertons and seven workers dead. With the Pinkerton agents unable to force the mill away from the workers, Frick turned to the National Guard, which sent in 8,500 men. These successfully took the town from the strikers and set up replacement workers to operate the mill. In a bit of targeted revenge, Frick was injured in a failed assassination attempt. On the other side, union leaders were indicted on a wide variety of charges from rioting to treason (Krause, 1992: 3–4). The strike dragged on from July to November, but in the end Frick was able to break the union as workers crossed the picket line and returned to work. Of the 3,800 strikers only 1,300 were permitted to work again, and none of them belonged to the union. Wages were reduced by an astonishing 50 percent, and extra Sunday pay abolished (Heilbroner, 1977: 136). Unionism in the national steel industry came to a halt for almost 40 years.

workforce, from the widespread use of spies to finger "problem" workers to shooting union leaders (Fitch, 1924: 177, 212). Firms would frequently hire agencies like Pinkertons or use their own private police to employ deadly tactics to intimidate workers. According to the Secretary of the Southern Industrial Convention, N. F. Thompson, "Labor organizations are ... the greatest menace to the government that exists .... [A] law should be passed that would make it justifiable homicide for any killing that occurred in defense of any lawful occupation" (cited in Heilbroner, 1977: 137).

Workers were not pacifists either. In 1877, the Pennsylvania Railroad buildings in Pittsburgh were burned down (Heilbroner, 1977: 46). In 1910 workers in California blew up the *Los Angeles Times* building because the company was one of the leaders of the open shop movement in the state (Weinstein, 1968: 173). Gunplay and fatalities were standard features of protest. What was also common was that the result of these violent conflicts most frequently went against the workers in the late nineteenth century (Dubofsky, 1996: 47).

As we saw in the Homestead strike, when employees appeared to be gaining the upper hand over their employers in industrial action, the state was quick to step in with either legislative or military aid for firms. In the recession of the 1890s, the US attorney-general in the Grover Cleveland administration, Richard Olney, authorized the use of government marshals and troops to break strikes across the United States, from a coal miners' strike in Indian territory to a transit strike in Minneapolis (Dubofsky, 1994: 29–30). As one scholar perceptively put it, the "state government and the army were simply the tools the owners used to combat an increasingly militant and active union movement" (Cooper, 1980: 170). The message to both employers and workers was clear. In the event of industrial conflict, firms could count on the military force of the state.

The use of physical force by the state was made possible by a legal system that was particularly one-sided in its ruling on labor matters. According to Dubofsky, "federal judges viewed strikes as disorderly by definition and as threats to the social order" (1994: 15). The law was used extensively to prevent the closed shop, picketing to prevent replacement workers, and boycotting the products of firms involved in industrial conflict, all of which are crucial weapons in the union armory. For both the judiciary and the state, worker activities in industrial conflicts were inevitably interpreted as signs of anarchy and insurrection that were direct challenges to the rule of law and order. They were also reviled as collusion and coercion, directly contradicting the right of employment of other workers. No matter what the rhetoric, the result was that by consistently lending the weight of the legal force of the state to employers, the government was actively creating conditions that kept wages low and living conditions poor. In fact, a better case could probably be made that state economic policy in support of private sector profits caused epidemic disease, than that it was caused by germs.

Ludlow

Sixteen years after the Homestead strike, there was yet another example of US industrial conflict escalating into small-scale warfare. The coal miners and owners of Colorado had a long history of nasty relations. Between 1903 and 1905 workers and private militia hired by the owners engaged in a running battle, featuring gunfights and dynamiting. State troopers attempted to quell the violence by predictably siding with the employers, instituting martial law and forcibly removing union leaders from the region. The grievances of the working population were hardly addressed by a repressive military crackdown, and simmered for years. After a major unionizing push in 1913, the United Mine Workers Union (UMW) approached the mining companies, the most important of which was Rockefeller-owned Colorado Fuel and Iron (CFI), demanding recognition of the union as bargaining agent, an eight-hour day, a 10 percent wage increase, ending the use of company script (money that could be used only at company-owned stores), elimination of armed guards, and the right to choose where to live. This list of demands, including as it does such basic rights as being paid in real money and choosing where to live, provides some indication of the conditions under which the miners were toiling. In the words of the federal mediator appointed to bring a resolution to the conflict, Ethelbert Stewart, the cause of the strike had its roots in the fact that miners were:

> prohibited from having any thought, voice or care in anything in life but work, and [were] assisted in this by gunmen whose function it was, principally, to see that you did not talk labor conditions with another man who might accidentally know your language—this was the contented, happy, prosperous condition

out of which this strike grew …. That men have rebelled grows out of the fact that they are men.

(PBS, 2000)

The attitude of CFI was well illustrated in a letter from the vice president, Lamont Bowers, to Rockefeller from October 1913:

Our net earnings would have been the largest in the history of the company by $200,000 but for the increase in wages paid the employees during the last few months. With everything running so smoothly and with an excellent outlook for 1914, it is mighty discouraging to have this vicious gang come into our state and not only destroy our profit but eat into that which has heretofore been saved.

(PBS, 2000)

In his testimony before Congress on April 6, 1914, Rockefeller gave some indication of the lengths to which he would go for the principle of the open shop: "we believe so sincerely that interest demands that the camps shall be open camps, that we expect to stand by the officers at any cost."

"And you will do that if it costs all your property and kills all your employees?"

"It is a great principle" (PBS, 2000).

The owners would not meet with the union representatives. Workers walked off the job in September 1913, and both sides started an arms build-up. The owners brought in an out-of-state militia, armed them with machine guns and dug them in around the mines as if for trench warfare. The union openly bought weapons for miners in a public warning to strike breakers (Weinstein, 1968: 192–3).

Predictably, violence flared quickly and escalated rapidly. Individual acts of violence and retaliation soon turned into pitched battles. The governor called in the National Guard to restore order, but this initially fairly neutral force was soon turned to protecting strike-breakers so that production in the mines could continue. Battles between the miners on one side, and the combination of private security and the National Guard on the other, escalated until the Guard attacked and then put a colony of striking miners to the torch, killing among others two women and eleven children. In response, the union called to arms every available miner and started to take over mines and towns in the region. They killed strike-breakers, dynamited mines, and set fire to mine buildings. Clearly unable to cope with such open warfare, the governor pleaded with President Wilson to send in the troops, which succeeded in restoring an uneasy peace (Weinstein, 1968: 194). The strike dragged on until December 1914, when the union was forced to call off the strike and tell members to return to work when they ran out of money.

While superficially the defeat at Ludlow appeared to be merely a repetition of the Homestead result, a closer examination reveals that Ludlow took place at a time that the government was being forced to reconsider its one-sided role in labor relations. An important indication of this was that Wilson instructed federal troops not to help owners use strike-breakers to continue production. The Ludlow conflict was also one of the events that led the United States to form a Commission on Industrial Relations (CIR), which produced a government document that was very sympathetic to the plight of US workers (Dubofsky, 1994: 57).

THE US TRANSFORMATION

Despite the repeated failures of worker resistance in the late 1800s and the almost complete destruction of several unions, in the early twentieth century, inequitable distribution of the gains from the economy led to further protests. Strikes were again prominent and were again violently put down. Yet during this period real gains were made, improving the lives of typical US residents. This section examines the political and economic changes that created an opportunity for US workers to gain, in a limited way, a more equitable share of the spoils from production, both in their work lives and the broader environment in which they lived.

Unlike Homestead, events such as Ludlow came at a time when increased worker organization and strength in the political system led to the gradual recognition that the groundswell of discontent had to be addressed. Although the events at Ludlow may have been more violent than the norm, industrial conflict and worker anger were obvious to any who were paying even the slightest attention. After the decimation of unions in the late 1800s, they grew rapidly in the first part of the twentieth century. In only seven years union membership increased from 447,000 in 1897 to 2,073,000 in 1904 (Dubofsky 1996: 102). This was not a period of labor peace. Annually, there were three times as many strikes in the early years of the twentieth century as there were in the late nineteenth (Dubofsky, 1996: 123).

There was also a change in union attitudes towards the political system during this period. Originally, unions were opposed to government regulation that intervened in the workplace in areas like minimum wages, maximum hours, and unemployment insurance, because they were concerned that regulation would decrease the role of unions, and because the legislative history of governments showed that they sided almost exclusively with business. Unions preferred to focus their energies on collective bargaining and the legal system. However, after a number of court defeats, in which judges consistently ruled in favor of business interests, unions began to reconsider their lack of engagement in the political process, so that by 1908 they started an increasingly close collaboration with the Democrats (Dubofsky, 1996: 108–9).

Political parties advocating a dramatic break from the current political economy were also growing in popularity. In the 1904 presidential election Eugene V. Debs quadrupled his vote running on a socialist platform. The socialist vote remained constant in 1908 and then surged again in 1911. Socialists were elected mayors in 73 municipalities in the United States (Weinstein, 1968: 118–20). The threat was deemed sufficiently grave that the leading organization of big businesses in the country, the National Civic Federation (NCF), conducted a sizeable campaign against the spread of socialism. After Wilson's 1912 election, the Democrats consciously adopted many pro-labor platforms in an attempt to woo voters away from socialist candidates (Dubofsky, 1996: 115).

The Progressive period started the improvements in people's lives that made for an increasingly inhospitable environment for infectious disease. Many of the reforms were championed by the large businesses of the NCF and implemented at the federal and state levels by the Democratic Party, but the only reason that these groups were interested in reform was the constant and often violent pressure from US workers. Essentially the movement for reform came about due to the recognition that the status quo of the late nineteenth century could not be sustained without the very real threat of growing mass discontent and continued pressure for much more widespread and radical change by workers (Weinstein, 1968: 13).

Poverty and inequality

During the early decades of the twentieth century there was a change in attitude towards the lot of the worker by those in positions of power in the United States. At the beginning of the period it was believed that poverty was the result of the failings of the individual. If workers were not paid enough it was because they had not obtained the skills or worked hard enough to earn a higher income. Protests, whether in unions or in the streets, were viewed as the anarchic grumblings of an undeserving mob attempting to ransom money from their betters. By the end of the period both government, and many of the larger employers represented by organizations like the NCF, recognized that without serious reform of the economic system, protest, often violent, would only intensify.

The federal government signaled a slight shift in its position by siding with workers on occasion. Wilson created a new Department of Labor, whose first secretary was a former official of the United Mine Workers. The federal government also passed a number of changes to national labor law, including the Clayton Act, which was designed to give unions some measure of protection from judicial rulings under the anti-monopoly or "anti-trust" Sherman Act (Dubofsky, 1996: 91). However, many of the changes were less the result of protective government regulation than they were a result of a combination of union pressure and what Dubofsky termed "welfare capitalism," which was the attempt by self-interested capitalists to limit turnover, absenteeism, and accidents, while reducing the threat of labor unrest, by improving the work lives of their employees (1996: 94). It was the threat of unions that forced employers into welfare capitalism.

Ford

Perhaps the most prominent example of welfare capitalism and the changes that were sweeping the nation during this period was Henry Ford's $5 day. While doubling his workers' daily wages understandably dominates the popular understanding of this move by Ford, it is less known that $2.66 of that was a bonus to be awarded upon meeting a number of criteria, and that at the same time he dropped the length of the day from nine to eight hours. Predictably such a drastic move demanded an explanation. The *Wall Street Journal* at the time argued that it was pure stupidity (Raff, 1988: 388). A more thoughtful reason is that it fitted nicely with welfare capitalism's attempts to reduce turnover, which was certainly a problem at Ford's plant. His switch from more artisanal production to the regimented routine of the assembly line created a turnover rate of 370 percent, with 39,000 resignations on a staff of 13,000 in 1913. By 1915, after the $5 day, turnover had dropped to 16 percent. However, while the high turnover prior to the $5 day was surely an inconvenience, 79 percent of the jobs at Ford could be mastered within a week, meaning that the cost of turnover was at most 16 percent of the wage increase (Raff, 1988: 392).

The second explanation was that Ford was paying an above-market wage to attract quality employees, and that their increased productivity would outweigh the growing wage bill. This explanation also has problems. With Ford's fancy new assembly line, the scope for discretion among workers was drastically reduced. Of course, this was one of the main advantages of the assembly line—to reduce the scope for highly skilled craft workers to control the pace and conditions of work. It also meant that jobs easily learned and mastered required very little in the way of high wages to motivate workers. The pace of work was set by the line. Further, there appeared to be few concerns at Ford with careless or shoddy work prior to the $5 day.

According to Harvard Business School Professor Daniel Raff, a more credible explanation is Ford's desire to prevent any industrial action or fledgling union activity. Ford was making far and away the most profit in the automobile industry. In 1913, Ford's profit of $27 million was over three times greater than the $8 million earned by General Motors in the same year. Ford's high profits meant that it was not sailing so close to the wind that it could not afford to throw some money to its workers. It also fueled workers' grievance about the distribution of income between the firm and its employees. Based on those profits (and a 51-week year), any work stoppage at Ford would have cost the company over $540,000 a week (Raff, 1988: 392). Further, the assembly line production at Ford made it especially vulnerable to collective action, especially a sit-down strike, where workers stop working and occupy the factory. In the broader context of industrial strife that we have seen in this period, Ford may have seen this as the largest threat to his lucrative operation. Joseph Galamb, the chief design engineer of the Model T, claimed that Ford instituted the $5 day to keep out the International Workers of the World (IWW), a radical union with the unimposing nickname of "the wobblies" (Raff, 1988: 398). According to Raff, the $5 day and the very real benefits that it generated for employees were due to Ford's desire to "buy the peace" (Raff, 1988: 399).

When the US Steel Corporation implemented its own workers' compensation program, its solicitor, Raynal Bolling, announced that it should serve as a "rebuke and rebuttal" to those who "assert that the workingmen get nothing except by contest and struggle" (cited in Weinstein, 1968: 47). According to Dubofsky, welfare capitalism was "basically intended to avert unionization" (1996: 97). Concessions by non-union firms were the workplace equivalent of the political reform movement in the sense that they offered some real concessions to the increasingly dissatisfied working class, but in a manner that was controlled by business.

US workers enjoyed stronger real wage gains after 1900. Recall from our introduction to the conditions in the last decades of the nineteenth century that real wages had grown 50 percent in the 40 years between 1850 and 1890, an average of 1.25 percent per year. Between 1890 and 1914 real wages increased 37 percent, an average of 1.54 percent per year (Dubofsky, 1996: 18). This understates the gains made after the turn of the century because this average is pulled down by very slow wage growth in the 1890s (Allen, 1994: 129–31). The upturn after about 1900 is especially pronounced for unskilled laborers, who were at the bottom end of the income spectrum, making them the most vulnerable portion of the population. An examination of six English-speaking cities in England, Canada, Australia, and the United States found that in 1880 San Francisco and Chicago were tied for the lowest real wage. Growth in wages for unskilled labor remained low until after 1900, when much stronger growth in the wages of unskilled workers moved US cities ahead of ahead of earlier industrializing cities like Manchester (Allen, 1994: 124).

Conditions of work

The combination of public protest, state involvement, and welfare capitalism also changed the conditions in which people worked. Many states restricted the kinds of jobs that could be held and the length of the work day for women and children (Rosen, 1958: 430), but governments at any level in the United States had little interest in regulating the hours of male workers, with the notable exception of the Adamson Act, which granted railway workers an eight-hour day, and some legislation in coal mining (Dubofsky, 1996: 91). However, a reduced work day became a fundamental principle of the American Federation of Labor (AFL) by 1886. It was secured in individual occupations by specific unions in the building trades in the late nineteenth century. As early as 1905, the eight-hour day was won in the printing trades, and in 1915 a series of successful strikes in the industrial centers of the United States that were gearing up for wartime production spread it more broadly. The length of the working day was also falling in non-union workplaces, as firms attempted to ward off the threat of unionization by providing some concessions to their employees.

The Triangle fire

The working conditions for the women in New York's clothing sweatshops were notoriously poor in the early twentieth century. Low wages, hazardous workplaces and long hours were the lot of the young, immigrant women who made up the bulk of the labor in this industry. In 1909, women at the Triangle Waist Company walked off the job in protest with the help of a middle-class women's group, the Women's Trade Union League (WTUL). Among the workers' demands were functioning fire escapes and open doors from the factories to the street (Davis, 1988: 4). The strike did not last long, and many of the organizers were dismissed for fomenting dissent. In response to the defeat, the International Ladies Garment Workers Union (ILGWU) organized a general strike by workers in the garment industry. Around 20,000 workers participated in a 13-week strike that succeeded in winning wage gains for around 15,000 workers—although the Triangle company was one of the holdouts that refused to recognize the union.

In 1911, the famous Triangle fire swept through the factory, killing 146 women and girls of the 500 workers in the shop. The factory was overcrowded and many of the horribly inadequate fire exits were locked (to prevent theft of materials), trapping workers inside the blaze. Unable to get out of the building, women were forced to jump from the ninth-floor windows in a doomed attempt to avoid being burned alive (Baxandall, Gordon, and Reverby, 1976: 202). Rose Schneiderman, vice president of the WTUL, placed the blame on the economic system that forced women to work in such hazardous conditions:

> The old Inquisition had its rack and thumb screws and its instruments of torture...We know what these things are today. The iron teeth are the necessities, the thumb screws the high powered and swift machinery close to which we must work, and the rack is here in the fire-trap structures that will destroy us.
>
> (cited in Rosner and Markowitz, 1997: 475)

The owners of Triangle, Isaac Harris and Max Blanck were charged with manslaughter in the second degree, because they locked the doors during working hours. However, a jury acquitted the pair because it could not conclude that the owners knew the doors were locked. Two years later, in 1913, Blanck was finally charged with locking one of the doors. He was fined $20 for the crime, "and the judge apologized to him for the imposition" (Cornell University ILR School, 2011).

The first steps were also taken to combat occupational hazards beyond fires and workers' compensation. At the turn of the century, a broad-based movement that included such unlikely collaborators as socialists, middle-class social reformers, and US Steel banded together in an effort to improve workplace health. These three groups had very different motivations. The socialists were looking to improve the lot of workers and use the horrid conditions of employment as a means to expose the exploitative conditions of early industrial capitalism. Middle-class reformers, like the Consumer League, were concerned that the poor working conditions were fostering diseases that could be transmitted through products, such as clothes, purchased by more affluent members of society. Employers were concerned that the high human costs were creating strong class antagonisms that, if unchecked, could only lead to more, stronger protests (Rosner and Markowitz, 1997: 473).

The Triangle fire (see the box) was an indictment of the conditions prevalent in the factories during the early twentieth century, but it also showed the new zeal to remedy these problems in the Progressive period. In the context of widespread public horror in the aftermath of the Triangle fire, unions in the garment trades like the ILGWU, and socially conscious women's reform movements like the WTUL, joined forces to successfully press for building codes that would prevent similar catastrophes by requiring fire extinguishers, alarms, unlocked fire doors, and hoses. The Factories Investigative Commission, appointed in response to the tragedy, took a much broader mandate to investigate the conditions in a wide range of trades, focusing not only on fire safety but also other issues from low wages to long hours. The Commission wrote over 30 changes to the state's labor laws, many of which were specifically targeted to protect women and children (Cornell University ILR School, 2011). The composition of the Commission also reflected the important role women played in driving progressive change. Among the 25-member commission were women such as Anne Morgan (niece of J. P. Morgan) and Frances Perkins, who was the head of the New York Consumers League. Perkins, who became secretary of labor during Roosevelt's New Deal Administration, declared that witnessing the fire galvanized her to dedicate her life to fighting for legislation that would improve the lives of US workers (Cornell University ILR School, 2011).

A wave of state-level workers' compensation regulations was passed to protect employees injured on the job during this period. In 1911 not a single state had legislation in this area, but by 1920 all but six (all in the South) had passed some form of compensation program. Program specifics varied considerably from state to state, but it is interesting to note that some states opted for state-run and financed programs while others went for a private insurance option. This was in contrast to the almost entirely government-provided systems of Europe. On the other hand, the government option went forward in many states despite the strong lobbying of the insurance industry, which attempted to brand the public option as socialist (Weinstein, 1968: 61).

Improvements in working conditions were brought about by a combination of union action, popular pressure, and legislative change. The AFL threw its weight behind the workplace safety movement. In one year the cloak makers union alone called 28 successful strikes over safety concerns in New York. Bakers also walked off the job, demanding better ventilation to combat high rates of tuberculosis. Government was pressured to overcome its reluctance to dictate the conditions of work. Between 1900 and 1910 state factory inspections were either created or expanded, health departments started to investigate occupational health concerns, and state acts regulated work in several specific industries such as tanneries, bakeries, and foundries (Rosner and Markowitz, 1997: 475–7). Factory codes were introduced requiring the removal of dust, and a prohibitive tax was placed on white phosphorus matches to stop the poisoning of workers (Rosen, 1958: 434). All these changes were symptomatic of a profound shift from the general belief highlighted earlier in the chapter, that injuries were either an accepted and inevitable part of work, or were the result of the worker's own negligence. By the end of this period it was generally acknowledged that society had the responsibility to guarantee a safe workplace (Rosner and Markowitz, 1997: 479).

Living conditions: housing, sanitation, and public health

As was the case in the United Kingdom, the Progressive period featured a concerted effort to improve the squalid urban environment. In fact, the "sanitation movement" was one of the forerunners of the Progressive movement. Epidemics of cholera and yellow fever, or even the threats of those diseases, created the spur for city improvements. The reaction by the wealthier members of society to the horribly poor and crowded living conditions that were breeding grounds for infectious disease took two forms. The most immediate, and selfish, was to move "up the hill" and away from the slums. However, this proved ineffective since the overcrowded cities were still a part of the urban environment of the middle classes before the automobile made the flight to the suburbs possible (Szreter, 2002b: 592). It was also too callous for many reform-minded individuals who were genuinely concerned with the lot of those less fortunate. It was a cholera scare that led to the creation of the New York Board of Health in 1866, which successfully reduced the death toll from a cholera epidemic the following year using an aggressive dual strategy of quarantine and sanitation. It was the concerns over disease outbreaks, especially the fears of epidemics, that created the successful push for a much broader role for the municipality in improving living conditions in the city in the late nineteenth and early twentieth century.

Across the country, popular pressure came from a diverse group of classes that banded together to lobby for municipal political solutions to public health issues. The pressure for reform in the wake of the Triangle fire was a microcosm of many of the alliances that were formed to advocate for change during this period. Much of the demand for reform came from workers and their allies in middle-class women's organizations. Under the name "municipal housekeeping," women declared their desire to clean up the entire city, a natural extension of their work within the home. Women were crucial in efforts to organize unions, promote sanitation, improve housing, abolish child labor, and create health programs for mothers and children (Fee, 1994: 234). These efforts were most often spearheaded by middle-class professionals like doctors or civil servants (Szreter, 2003: 425), and supported by both the lower-income members of the working class, who were the most direct beneficiaries, and their more affluent middle-income colleagues, creating a "collective responsibility for inner cities" (Szreter, 2002b: 592). The commitment to urban improvements among the upper and middle-income groups was sufficiently strong that they agreed to increased taxes on their property and wealth in order to finance these changes (Szreter, 2003: 425).

It was this period that saw dramatic improvements in sewage disposal, safe water supplies, clean streets, and pure milk for the children of the poor (Duffy, 1997: 424). In 1875, filtered water was only available to around 30,000 urbanites. By 1910, that number had increased an astonishing 333-fold to 10 million, which was still only 25 percent of the urban population (Meeker, 1974: 392). Public health programs not only included infrastructure projects, but also extended to food inspections and maternity services. Philadelphia, for example, implemented a wide variety of public health programs by 1914, from children's health clinics to regulating the milk supply, which was notoriously adulterated and improperly handled, especially in low-income areas (Condran, Williams, and Cheney, 1997: 459–64).

Economic historian Edward Meeker attempted the challenging task of quantifying the benefits from public health investment between 1880 and 1910 (although this was done as early as 1873, when Pettenkofer published "The value of health to a city," which estimated that the benefits of public sanitation in Munich would vastly outweigh its costs: Evans, 1973: 169). The benefits were defined very narrowly as reduction of work time lost because of eight diseases, and the value of increasing life expectancy. These benefits were compared with the costs of sewers, water filtration, and spending on health conservation and maintenance, such as smallpox vaccines. Meeker concluded that, at its very lowest, the social rate of return was between 6 and 16 percent, considerably above the return on private investments such as bonds or the railroads. Even on narrow economic grounds, in which many of the benefits of public health are not counted, the investment quite literally paid off (Meeker, 1974: 417). The motive to improve the worst of the urban living conditions stemmed from a combination of compassion and self-preservation on the part of the middle classes. Yet, these measures represented an acknowledgement that it was a combination of low incomes and lack of public services, both characteristics of this early stage of industrial capitalism in the United States, that were responsible for epidemic conditions. If poverty was not eliminated, at least the dearth of municipal infrastructure was.

CONCLUSION

The United States is not identical to the United Kingdom. Unlike the United Kingdom, the United States had a more positive experience with early-stage industrial capitalism. It appears as though incomes grew on average more steadily in the United States, whereas the United Kingdom experienced an extensive stagnation. However, there were some very real growing pains in the United States as well. Income was still unhealthily low for many, below what contemporary observers considered a bare subsistence wage. As was the case in the United Kingdom, the conditions in which people worked and lived made them very susceptible to infectious disease. This poverty was caused not only by an overall low level of income created by the economy, but by how that income was distributed. These conditions were the inevitable result of firms attempting to lower their labor costs and equipment expenses, but they were also caused by the government serving as what a Marxist might call "the instrument of capital." Both the political and judicial arms of the state acted time and again to suppress the claims of workers and support those of capital. This was true when troops were used to ensure that replacement workers could safely be used to break strikes, and when workers were denied compensation for injuries in the courts. Infectious disease was prominent when political and economic structures favored capital at the expense of labor so blatantly that it left a large portion of the working population virtually at death's door.

Only when these conditions started to change was epidemic disease conquered in the United States. These changes were not simply the result of economic growth and productivity gains. Economic growth was only channeled to working-class incomes, civic improvements and better working conditions when the populace became sufficiently mobilized that they created pressure for a redistribution of the income earned by society towards these purposes. It was protest from labor that created a more livable workday and a higher wage. It was pressure from a broad coalition of citizens that brought about safer workplaces and more healthy cities. It was these improvements, drawing from emerging public health knowledge, that conquered infectious disease in the United States, not a medical miracle.

4

DEATH IN OUR TIMES: THE EXCEPTIONAL CLASS CONTEXT FOR CHRONIC DISEASE IN THE UNITED STATES

> ... health inequalities result from the differential accumulation of exposures and experiences that have their sources in the material world ... the effect of income inequality on health reflects a combination of negative exposures and lack of resources held by individuals, along with systematic under investment across a wide range of human, physical, health, and social infrastructure.
>
> (Lynch et al., 2000: 1202)

In Bill Bryson's entertaining guide to the sciences, *A Short History of Nearly Everything* (2003), one of his scientific hero figures was Iowa farm boy Clair Patterson. Not only did Patterson manage to successfully determine the age of the Earth in 1953, he also spearheaded the battle against the use of lead. Bryson's villain in the lead story was Thomas Midgley, who pioneered the use of lead in gasoline (and just for good, damaging, measure also discovered chlorofluorocarbons—CFCs) to reduce engine knock while working for General Motors (GM) in 1923. Realizing a valuable substance when it saw one, GM banded together with DuPont and Standard Oil to form the Ethyl Corporation, with the goal of getting as much lead into products as people could possibly buy. Lead was sprayed on fruit, used in food tins, and appeared in toothpaste tubes. As we now know, lead is a neurotoxin.

Exposure to lead, even in small doses, damages the brain and central nervous system. It is associated with blindness, kidney failure, and cancer, among other health issues. Health concerns were first noticed in workers producing lead, although at the time the spokesman for Ethyl claimed that "These men probably went insane because they worked too hard" (Bryson, 2003: 150). Repeated denials, expensive public relations campaigns, industry-funded junk science, and legal actions served the lead industry well. As late as 2001 the Ethyl Corporation stated "that research has failed to show that leaded gasoline poses a threat to human health or the environment." Despite overwhelming evidence of the dangers of lead, much of which was pioneered by Patterson in the face of considerable industry pressure, the sale of leaded gasoline did not end in the United States until 1986. Lead solder was not banned from food containers until 1993, and indoor lead paint was used for 40 years in the United States after it was banned in most of Europe. Although the level of lead in people's blood has fallen by 80 percent in the United States since 1986, because lead never really disappears they still have 625 times the lead levels of people living a hundred years ago (Bryson, 2003: 154–6). This is not a story about the particular greed of one company. Rather, it is the story of modern capitalism, especially in its exceptional US form.

The conditions that fostered infectious disease were alleviated through a combination of an organized working-class resistance and broader social movements. Working-class demands led to improvements in wages (and therefore food, housing, and clothing), reduced work hours, and child labor laws. Broader social coalitions of professionals, middle-class reformers, and workers won urban improvements such as clean water and sanitation. However, in the economic world of the firm these victories have a cost. In the absence of increases in productivity, increasing benefits for a firm's employees will inevitably decrease profits. Rising wages and profits are only possible with accompanying increases in productivity, or getting more value out of each hour of labor. The transformation from making profits by "squeezing" labor to making profits by increasing worker productivity is the evolution from absolute to relative surplus value in capitalism. According to Marx, "relative surplus-value functions through revolutionizing the technical processes of labor and the groupings into which society is divided" (1967 [1867]: 645).

Firms that were able to introduce techniques that lowered unit labor costs under these conditions would make more profits that they could invest in new techniques to stay ahead in the race that is capitalist competition. This dynamic decreased the labor time needed to make products through productivity increases. These investments made possible, although not inevitable, growing wages and benefits for workers. This is, after all, the genius of capitalism:

its laws of motion generate economic growth. But growth is unstable, generating recessions and depressions. The very same profit-maximizing dynamic also creates an incentive to offload the costs of production from the private to the public system, disproportionally affecting the health and well-being of its majority working population.

This increase in productivity took place primarily through mechanization. In the twentieth century, mechanization for cost-minimizing, profit-maximizing capitalist firms has tended to generate a more energy- and chemical-intensive production process, which in turn has resulted in significant changes in the environment in which people live and the products that they consume. This marks an historically significant transformation, particularly with respect to the context for disease. In part, this transformation led to the productivity/wage increases that made possible improvements in health and the decline in the effects of infectious diseases. However, in the hands of cost-minimizing/profit-maximizing capitalists, this transformation also resulted in the creation of the "age of chronic disease." Thus, overcoming infectious disease came at a price. By introducing more mechanized/intensive production processes, capitalism transformed the context for disease. It has transformed our food, water, air and work processes in unprecedented ways, and created the historically unique disease pattern that we identified as being so stubbornly immune to mainstream medical interventions in Chapter 2. According to Lester Breslow, former director of public health for the state of California and UCLA professor of public health, "With all due respect to genetics and to theories that attribute chronic disease to senescence, it would be more rewarding to examine the changes that have occurred over the past half century in man's diet, habits, forms of work, and physical surroundings" (cited in Dubos, 1965: 287).

These broad changes have occurred in all industrial nations, but as we shall demonstrate here and in Chapter 6, the United States has done less to counter the negative impacts brought on by these changes than other nations. As we mentioned in Chapter 1, the broad health indicators in the United States, such as life expectancy and infant mortality, are among the worst in the industrialized world. The United States was ranked fourth highest out of 34 countries in potential life years lost through premature death (OECD, 2011: 27). Its record on heart disease and cancer is not much better. According to the OECD, in 2011 the United States ranked tenth highest out of the 34 countries for ischemic heart disease mortality. Most of the countries with higher rates than the United States were Eastern European countries such as Poland, Russia, and the Czech Republic (OECD, 2011: 29) The United States had the seventh highest rate of overall cancer incidence out of 40 nations in 2011 (although it fares much better in terms of cancer mortality rates) (OECD, 2011: 31, 45). In some ways, like its low smoking rate, the United States is doing reasonably well, yet the high US ranking in heart disease mortality, cancer rates, and life years lost reinforces the point that US health is not what it could be.

An exhaustive review of the tidal wave of change in the products that we consume and the manner in which they are produced would be impossible. In the sections that follow we will look at some important examples of recent changes (to food, the environment, work, and social stratification) that illustrate the strength of the political economy approach in explaining the current pattern of chronic disease in industrialized countries. Although this chapter is divided into these sections for the sake of organization, it is important to remember that many of the issues cross these neat divisions. For example, pesticides sprayed on crops create health risks at work for agricultural laborers in the field, for the environment when they run into rivers and lakes, and at the table when families eat their daily greens. All of these examples stress the importance of economic, political, and social reality in creating the diseases that currently kill most people.

FOOD

Food production has undergone a remarkable transformation. The industrialization of agriculture has had important benefits. Yields and productivity have increased dramatically with the introduction of scientific techniques into food production. This has allowed much more food to be produced, at a lower cost, so that the Malthusian concern about population outpacing food production has been, at least thus far, staved off. The cost advantages of large industrial operations (now there is a name for them in animal farming—concentrated animal feeding operations or CAFOs) over smaller farms have resulted in a dramatic change in agriculture away from the romantic version of the family farm toward large-scale production (MacDonald and McBride, 2009). However, the introduction of new techniques and technology into the food production system has had some problematic consequences for human health. For example, fat has been qualitatively transformed and its intake in this century has increased both absolutely and as a proportion of our food consumption. We are eating more saturated fats, those most dangerous to the coronary arteries (Walker et al., 2005). The food industry has transformed the old type of animal fats into a new type, which is remarkably efficient at increasing the cholesterol in our blood (Blumenfeld, 1964: 123).

The food industry transformed our daily food, creating a mixture with a high proportion of saturated fat that boosts cholesterol, because it was less expensive to keep cattle in a stall, away from exercise, making it easier to feed and fatten them, than to allow cattle to roam the range. Instead of eating grass and slowly growing into marketable animals, cattle are fed grains (mostly corn, which is even fed to fish, thanks to generous US government subsidies to corn farmers) spiked with chemicals. This results in marbled steak, which affects the quality of the meat. Not only does marbled steak have a higher fat content, this process of "producing cattle" changes the partially unsaturated fats into a hard, white, much more saturated fat (Pollan, 2002a). In the days when there were "free range" hogs, scientists used lard as a source of unsaturated fats in laboratory experiments. Rooting for food meant soft and unsaturated lard, but "scientifically" fed hogs become extremely heavy hogs whose lard becomes supersaturated fat. In most large operations, hens no longer "free range" for worms, insects, seeds, and grass. The priming of hens means restricted movement by housing them in cubicles while feeding them scientific mixtures designed to produce the maximum number of eggs per day—regardless of their quality. The results are abnormal eggs with supersaturated fat, loaded with just the type of fats to be avoided at all costs in an anticoronary diet (Blumenfeld, 1964: 125).

Even vegetarians who avoid cows, chickens, and hogs will not be spared the adverse health consequences of modern agriculture. In this age of processed foods, vegetable oil has become a ubiquitous feature of our diets. Industrial chemists have changed unsaturated vegetable oils into a new and most objectionable artificially saturated vegetable oil found in baked goods, fried food, and snacks. In order to extend the shelf life of oil, food manufacturers hydrogenate vegetable oils. This process hardens the oil into a synthetic hard solid fat, which will not spoil, and it is a major contributor to coronary disease. The negative health impacts of transfats have been sufficiently well demonstrated that some cities (New York, Philadelphia) and states (California) have banned it in restaurants.

Visual appeal is crucial for food sales, but often comes at the expense of quality. Fruits are picked before they are ripe and gassed as they are transported across country so that they may appear ready to eat. In this way, green tomatoes become ripe without companies needing to wait for them to ripen or spoiling in transit or on the shelf. Similarly, artificial food coloring and flavoring makes food appear to have the qualities that people want and at lower cost. For example, food coloring is used to make oranges more orange. The bright colors made possible by dyes are especially popular in food targeted at children. Over 17 million pounds of food dyes were produced in the United States in 2005 for goods as diverse as candy, baked goods, and beverages. Of the seven food dye colors permitted in the United States in 2005, two were banned in the European Union, three others banned in Norway and one other prohibited in France and Finland (Public Citizen Health Research Group, 1985). The prevalence of food additives like dyes comes despite nagging worries among many in the scientific community that they have links to cancer. One review of the literature claims that "artificial dyes may be involved in chemical induced carcinogenesis due to their mutagenic properties" (Irigaray et al., 2007: 651).

The transition of food production into a technologically advanced industry has meant that agriculture firms have applied increasingly scientific techniques in an effort to produce more food, more cheaply. Unfortunately, some of these techniques have been linked to cancer-causing agents. Carcinogens in food include growth hormones (such as Carbadox, used in pork production, and Revlar, used in beef production) and nitrites used in preserved meats such as hot dogs to keep them looking pink and fresh longer. The nitrites combine with amines, which are naturally present in the meat to form N-Nitrosodimethylamine, classified by the International Agency for Research on Cancer (IARC) as a probable human carcinogen. Studies have linked consumption of hot dogs more than once per week to increased brain cancers and leukemia in children. Children whose mothers ate hot dogs more than once per week while they were pregnant have also been found to have increased rates of cancer (Epstein, 1998: 574–6).

The same large-scale industrial production and government subsidies (a 2002 farm bill set aside $4 billion a year for ten years for corn growers) that make corn the preferred animal feed also make corn syrup a cheaper sweetener than sugar, a fact that has not gone unnoticed by the snack food and beverage industry. By the turn of the twenty-first century 10 percent of the calories in the US diet came from corn sweeteners. For children the figure was closer to 20 percent (Pollan, 2002b). A growing intake of corn syrup has been linked most commonly to increasing rates of obesity, but also to kidney disease (Shoham et al., 2008) and liver disease (Ouyang et al., 2008).

All of these problems are exacerbated by how food is consumed in the United States. As we show later in the chapter, people are living increasingly stressful lives, often on relatively meager budgets. This has created an opportunity for the dramatic expansion of the fast-food industry in the country. The astounding calorie count in a quick, cheap meal consisting of a burger, shake, and fries is unlikely to reduce the problems of heart disease and obesity. Yale professor of public health Kelly Brownell is especially critical of the role that fast-food companies play in creating what he calls, a "toxic food environment" (Brownell, 1998). According to the *New York Times,* in the late 1990s 7 percent of the US population was eating at McDonald's every day. One of the food chain's goals is to cover the country so that no one is ever more than four minutes away from a Happy Meal—presumably by car (Brownell, 1998).

Of course, the debate rages about what to do about gluttonous food consumption. The medical profession looks for the "fat" gene or drugs to manage weight. The behavioralists institute programs such as "Shape Up America" to convince people to change their unhealthy ways. While both of these approaches have some merit, they cannot really explain why obesity has increased so dramatically since the 1980s. It is unlikely that the genetic composition of people in the United States has changed in such a short span of time. It seems only slightly more possible that people have less willpower than 30 years ago, or are increasingly keen on lifestyle choices that predictably result in bigger tummies and heart attacks. A far better explanation is that firms have become ever more adept at convincing an increasingly budget- and time-constrained populace that a quick, easy, cheap, unhealthy meal really is what they want. As Brownell claims, "This is capitalism at its best" (1998).

The link between diet and chronic disease has been well established. Studies have found that the Mediterranean diet, containing less meat and more fruits and vegetables than the "Anglo" diets of North America and the United Kingdom, is associated with increased life expectancy and less illness. Unfortunately, people in the Mediterranean nations have been changing their eating habits to more closely resemble the Anglo diet. For example, Italians consumed 500 more calories per day in 1992 than they did in 1961, mostly because of a rise in high fat intake, from 25 to 39 percent of total calories. As a result, Italians are starting to succumb to the mortality patterns found in the United States (Dubois, 2006: 141). In the United States, changes in diet have had conflicting effects on health. On one hand, the reduction in cholesterol has contributed to a decline in coronary heart disease. However, this beneficial effect is being partially offset by the negative impact of the increase in the body-mass index of the US population (Ford et al., 2007: 2,395).

Given the link between diet and chronic disease, recent trends in US food consumption have experts concerned about an obesity "epidemic." Since the 1990s, total calories, saturated fat, and absolute fat consumption in the United States have all increased rapidly for both adults and children (Dubois, 2006: 142). As always, these broad trends vary for different groups in society. For example, higher-income groups have healthier diets (for similar reasons that they have less stress and live longer lives, discussed later in the chapter) and males displayed stronger improvements in decreasing fat as a percent of total calories than women (Dubois, 2006: 143). Yet the overall trend is unquestionable and very concerning insofar as there are health risks associated with being overweight.

The health problems related to food are the result of a complex array of factors. No one is denying the importance of eating right and the fortune of a good genetic make-up. Yet, the economics of modern food production and consumption in the United States have contributed to some major health problems, which are not inevitably correlated with advances in agricultural productivity but are determined by the profit motive and class-based differences in consumption.

ENVIRONMENT

As crude a weapon as the cave man's club, the chemical barrage has been hurled against the fabric of life a fabric on the one hand delicate and destructible, on the other miraculously tough and resilient, and capable of striking back in unexpected ways. These extraordinary capacities of life have been ignored by the practitioners of chemical control who have brought to their task no high-minded orientation, no humility before the vast forces with which they tamper.

(Rachel Carson, 1964: 297)

New production techniques have also resulted in a bewildering array of substances, many of which are relatively recently invented and whose health impacts are not well understood, being released into the environment. This is inevitable in an economic system that is driven by profit-enhancing innovation. It is also inevitable that profit-maximizing firms will attempt to minimize the costs that they themselves incur in eliminating the dangers presented by these substances. This has given rise to a wide variety of health problems associated with modern capitalist production, from the local dangers of famously polluted sites such as the Love Canal (Niagara Falls, New York), to hazards associated with specific products like lead, to those that travel far and wide like airborne pollutants.

Local environmental problems affect small groups of people very intensely, and they are more common than most people think. The US Congressional Office of Technology Assessment estimates that there are 439,000 abandoned waste sites in the country (Davis, 2007: 340). Approximately 41 million people live within four miles of a superfund site (the Environmental Protection Agency (EPA) program set up to deal with hazardous waste). People living close to superfund sites have elevated risks of an ominous array of diseases including heart disease, genital malformations, childhood leukemia, hyperactivity, central nervous system damage, and Hodgkin's disease (Faber and Krieg, 2002: 279).

Local environmental problems are not distributed evenly across income groups. It is most often the less affluent members of the working class who live in hazardous proximity to these kinds of dangers. This result has been found in many different countries. In the United Kingdom, communities were ranked from poorest to richest and assessed for the number of unfavorable environmental conditions in each area (see Figure 4.1). Over 20 percent of the poorest communities contained three or more problematic conditions and only 28 percent had none. In contrast, 71 percent of the richest areas had no adverse environmental conditions and none had three or more (Marmot, 2010: 25).

Similar results are found in the United States. Louisiana is the poorest state in the union. It is famously home to "Cancer Alley," a 150-mile stretch between Baton Rouge and New Orleans that has 150 petrochemical and chemical facilities. It also has the highest cancer mortality rate in the United States (Katz 2012: 102). Another study ranked the environmental hazards from a wide variety of industrial sources in 368 communities in Massachusetts. All but one of the 15 most "intensively burdened towns" had an average household income of under $40,000. There was also a pronounced racial gradient. Only 20 towns in Massachusetts had a non-white population of over 15 percent. Yet of these 20 towns, nine were among the 15 most burdened. The study concludes that "the communities most heavily burdened with environmentally hazardous industrial facilities and sites are overwhelmingly low-income towns and/or communities of color" (Faber and Krieg 2002: 286).

Environmental problems can also spread over a much wider area. According to the American Cancer Society (ACS), although 80 percent of cancers in the United States are caused by "environmental" (as opposed to hereditary) factors, only 2 percent of these can be attributed to environmental pollutants (ACS, 2010: 50). However, this estimate (and that of occupational causes of cancer) has been called "woefully out of date"—the result of a decades-old study, rife with methodological problems (Reuben, 2010: 2). Linking specific pollutants or chemicals to particular diseases is complex (a point to which we return later in the chapter). As a result most of the links are still only theories. For example, it is true that women who begin menstruating before the age of 12 have a 30 percent greater

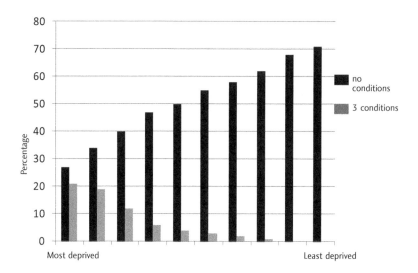

Figure 4.1 Percentage of neighborhoods with negative environmental conditions* by income decile, United Kingdom, 2010

* Environmental conditions: poor scores for river water quality, air quality, green space, habitat favorable to biodiversity, flood risk, litter, detritus, housing conditions, road accidents, regulated sites (e.g. landfill).

Source: Marmot (2010: 25).

chance of breast cancer than those who begin after the age of 15. It is also true that on average in the year 1800 US women began menstruating at the age of 17. In 2010 the average age was 12. However, discovering the precise reason for this change is difficult. One theory points to endocrine disrupters found in plastics and cosmetics, which are similar to estrogen and may set off early hormonal changes (Kristof, 2009).

A recent paper makes the reasonable point that although the links for cancer are sufficiently complex that attempting to estimate the percentage of any particular cancer caused by any individual source might be unwise and counterproductive, this should not prevent society from acting to minimize workplace and environmental causes of cancer (Clapp, How, and Lefevre, 2005: 632). To provide just one example from the United States, a survey of 500,000 people showed a connection between cancer rates and air pollution. Residents in areas with the worst air pollution are about 30 percent more likely to develop lung cancer than those in cities with clean air (Davis, 2007: 229). Similarly, children in high traffic areas have higher rates of leukemia (Irigaray et al., 2007: 648). The specific connection has not yet been identified in these cases. Yet this does not mean that society should not strive for less polluted air.

Identifying the specific connection between one kind of chemical, or perhaps even a combination of chemicals and health risks, is very challenging. In part, this is because of the complex interaction between a growing list of environmental pollutants, and evidence that suggests that the connections between different contaminants "may have synergistic effects that intensify or otherwise alter their impact compared with the effect of each contaminant alone" (Reuben, 2010: 2). It is also because detecting the environmental links to cancer has been given a very low funding priority, especially compared with genetic links to cancer. In 2008, only 14 percent of the National Cancer Institute (NCI) budget was spent on occupational or environmental research (Reuben, 2010: 5). As a result, exposures to cancer-causing agents and the manner in which different contaminants interact remain virtually unstudied.

Chapter 2 showed that the age-adjusted incidence of cancer is increasing, suggesting that the recent growth in cancer rates must be caused by changes found outside "naturally" occurring factors. It is also true that a large number of chemicals that cause tumors in animals are in widespread production in the United States. At least 29 of these chemicals are produced in quantities of at least 1 million pounds per year. Of these, most, like vinyl chloride, are found in consumer products. Others, like 1,2-dibromomethane are air pollutants. Many, of course, are both (Davis, 2007: 288). The IARC investigated 880 industrial substances between 1972 and 2003 to determine the likelihood that they were carcinogenic. It classified 89 of these as definite, a further 64 to be likely and another 264 as possible carcinogens (Clapp, Howe, and Jacobs, 2007: 638). Studies have linked increases in prostrate, kidney, testis, and breast and lung cancers to increased exposure to industrial chemicals (Faber and Krieg, 2002: 279). Here are a couple of examples of carcinogenic chemicals in everyday products (for a much more exhaustive list see Katz, 2012: 98–100):

The herbicide 2,4-D has been classified by the IARC as a possible human carcinogen. One of the brands of 2,4-D is sold in the United States as some forms of Roundup®, manufactured by Monsanto. Monsanto also sells "Roundup Ready"® seeds for canola, soybeans, and other crops, promoted as "genetically modified to be tolerant to in-crop applications of Roundup® herbicide."

Some cosmetics contain carcinogens including DEA (diethanolamine), formaldehyde and talc contaminated with asbestos. Women in particular are at risk, since they tend to use more lotions and cosmetics than men. Long-term use of permanent hair-coloring

The President's Cancer Panel

A 2010 report by the President's Cancer Panel expressed concern over the influence of chemicals on cancer rates. Both the number of new chemicals and the extent to which these have been tested for safety are worrying. Every year between 1–2,000 new chemicals are created and introduced into industrial processes. "Only a few hundred of the more than 80,000 chemicals in use in the United States have been tested for safety" (Reuben, 2010: ii). To the extent that there is a lack of evidence on the links between chemicals and cancer, it might be because of a lack of investigation rather than a lack of impact.

The panel also criticized US regulatory oversight of chemicals: U.S. regulation of environmental contaminants is rendered ineffective by five major problems: 1) inadequate funding and insufficient staffing, 2) fragmented and overlapping authorities coupled with uneven and decentralized enforcement, 3) excessive regulatory complexity, 4) weak laws and regulations, and 5) undue industry influence.

Source: Reuben (2010: ii).

products has been linked to an increased risk of bladder cancer and adult acute leukemia among both users and the hairdressers who apply these chemicals (Irigaray et al., 2007: 648–52).

Without downplaying the very real lifestyle factors associated with cancer such as obesity, alcohol, and smoking, it is clear that these are not sufficient explanations for current cancer trends. Many cancers that have not been linked to alcohol and tobacco are on the rise. In addition, other cancers, like renal cell carcinoma, that have been linked to these factors are also rising despite the decline in alcohol and tobacco use in many countries. The link between obesity and cancer might not be the result of obesity in itself, but because of build-up of chemical carcinogens in the adipose tissue. Similarly the link between aging and cancer might not be merely an inevitable result of the aging process, but rather reflect prolonged, increased exposure to chemical agents (Irigaray et al., 2007: 643–7). To rule out environmental factors is to ignore the obvious when a shockingly long list of industrial materials has been linked to cancer. Radiation has been linked to leukemia, lymphoma, thyroid cancer, breast cancer, and skin cancer. Air pollution like nitrogen dioxide has been linked to lung cancers. Indoor air is often polluted with volatile organic compounds like benzene and 1,3 butadiene that the IARC has ranked carcinogenic.

Many pesticides are rated as possibly carcinogenic, are endocrine disrupters and are strong immunosuppressors. Parental exposure (and direct exposure) to pesticides has been linked to childhood cancers including leukemia. Prolonged exposure to dioxins is linked with increased risk of cancer. Exposure to metals such as chromium, nickel, arsenic oxide, lead, mercury, and cadmium is linked to increases in cancer rates. Medicines and beauty products contain carcinogens.

In a telling illustration of the ubiquitous nature of chemicals in our environment, PBS journalist Bill Moyers and eight other volunteers were tested for the presence of chemicals, pollutants, and pesticides in their blood and urine. None of the volunteers worked in jobs that would obviously place them at risk of contamination or worked with chemicals on the job, yet they had an average of 91 compounds in their bodies, most of which did not even exist 75 years ago. More worryingly, on average 53 of the chemicals were linked to cancer in humans or animals (Environmental Working Group, 2003). In addition, studies have shown that more chemicals are found in women than in men (Reuben, 2010: 26).

The precise health effects of carrying around these chemicals are not really known, making the ACS proclamations of the limited effect of environmental factors even more speculative than most estimates of this type. When illness is caused by these kinds of environmental problems, the genetic and behavioral explanations carry even less weight. While some genetics may make people more susceptible to environmental problems, it is clear that they are

---

Obesity and chemicals

The major environmental influence on birth weight has been considered to be in utero nutrition. Therefore, maternal nutrition has been the focus of research into the fetal basis of diseases including obesity. However, nutrition is not the only environmental influence that may have an effect on adult diseases. There is increasing evidence that in utero exposure to environmental chemicals at environmentally relevant concentrations may alter developmental programming via alterations in gene expression or gene imprinting that do not result in either low birth weight or malformations but in functional deficits that do not become apparent until later in life where they surface as increased susceptibility to disease .... These data suggest a role for toxicology in the etiology of obesity. This role has received additional support from a recent review (Baillei-Hamilton, 2002) that presents a provocative hypothesis to explain the global obesity epidemic: chemical toxins. This article presents data showing that the current epidemic in obesity cannot be explained solely by alterations in food intake and/or decrease in exercise. There is a genetic predisposition component of obesity; however, genetics could not have changed over the past few decades, suggesting that environmental changes might be responsible for at least part of the current obesity epidemic. Indeed, the level of chemicals in the environment is purported to coincide with the incidence of obesity, and examples of chemicals that appear to cause weight gain by interfering with elements of the human weight control system—such as alterations in weight-controlling hormones, altered sensitivity to neurotransmitters, or altered activity of the sympathetic nervous system—are noted. Indeed, many synthetic chemicals are actually used to increase weight in animals.

Source: Heindel (2003).

not the cause. It is also difficult to see how people are choosing environmental pollution as a "lifestyle" choice. Environmental dangers that lurk in the areas in which they live are rarely known, and even if they are suspected, the only real solution is either the individually uprooting option of moving, or the difficult collective response of changing the political and economic rules that makes the pollution possible. Dangers associated with particular products could be avoided if they are known, but as the controversy around the safety of bisphenol A demonstrates, often they are not known, nor are the risks particularly well understood. Environmental risks highlight most obviously the importance of political and economic factors in determining public health.

WORK

The idea that people love to work would be hotly contested by those who grudgingly trudge off to their despised job every weekday morning. Yet, humans do love to work. Most people spend their off work hours happily engaging in a variety of pursuits from mountain climbing to gardening that require a great deal of what would be commonly thought of as "work." Of course, the difference between people dedicating their leisure time to growing potatoes and an agricultural worker toiling away on a large farm is the conditions under which work is done. Paid employment is the principal method by which the vast majority of the population not fortunate enough to have large inheritances "earn their corn," as the British say. This alone would grant it a central place in people's lives, since it is labor income that determines our ability to consume. Yet work is more than a mere cash transaction, it is also the place where most people spend a large portion of their lives. It is the place where people derive a considerable amount of their identity and their social esteem. It is where most people's dreams are either realized or thwarted, and is therefore where most people derive satisfaction and experience frustration. Given the centrality of work in people's lives it is unsurprising that it has a profound impact on health, beyond even its role in determining income. The conditions of modern work influence chronic disease in a variety of ways. As was the case with environmental factors, the relationship between work and disease is very complicated but we have divided the impacts into three categories: work stress, job insecurity, and old-fashioned occupational illness.

Stress at work

Negative health results appear more frequently for those at the lower end of the labor spectrum. For example, in contrast to popular belief, stress is not an executives' disease, despite the supposed pressure at the top of the corporate hierarchy. In fact, stress exists in higher proportions among the lower echelons of organizations (Evans, 1994: 13). In the now famous Whitehall study of British civil servants, those in higher positions had significantly better health results than those lower down the hierarchy. What makes this study particularly interesting is that none of the people in the study could be considered "poor" in any absolute sense of the word. They all had sufficient incomes to afford medical care, healthy housing and nutritious diets. Few, if any, worked in what would be called dangerous jobs. Yet the coronary mortality of those in the lower ranks (clerical and manual) was three and a half times that of those in the top levels (Rose and Marmot, 1981). This difference in mortality persists even when obvious differences in causes of death, like smoking, body mass index, and cholesterol, are accounted for. As a very interesting rebuttal to the behavioral school, the study found that those at lower pay grades smoked more than those at top grades (which in itself calls for an explanation), and that those in the higher echelons who did smoke were much less likely to contract smoking-related diseases than those lower down. So there is something about people's position in the labor market that influences health results beyond either being poor or making particular lifestyle choices.

One of the explanations devised to explain the connection between work hierarchy and stress is the demand–control model, in which stress increases in work situations where people face high psychological demands but have limited decision-making power (Marmot, Siegrist, and Theorell, 2006: 101). Evidence suggests that those who can make decisions actually have less stress, while those who have less autonomy over their work life generate increased adrenal hormones and fat energy. A clerk, stuck in a stressful routine, who is subject to the authority of someone else suffers from a very different sort of stress from an executive who has too many appointments in a day but who exercises significant authority (Karasek and Theorell, 1990). Stress hormones can make the blood "sticky" and may eventually over long periods of time degrade the immune system, make tumors grow faster and harden the arteries (Epstein, 1998). In a more active time in our evolution, stress hormones were used for "fight or flight" purposes; now they help create deposits such as plaque in the internal linings of the arteries. High-demand and low-control jobs have been linked to increases in coronary heart disease, as well as increased incidence of psychological strain and more minor illness, even when the classic "behavioral" factors are accounted for (Marmot et al., 2006: 107).

The second explanation is known as the effort–reward model. This associates work stress with high-effort–low-reward conditions. Rewards can either be in the most obvious form of wages or in other less tangible forms like recognition. When people work in conditions in which they feel they are putting in a great deal of effort and receiving little reward, this violates a sense of what is "fair" in society, creating considerable stress. Jobs that rank high on an effort-to-reward scale are associated with a variety of poor health results, but are most strongly associated with increased incidence of coronary heart disease, especially among middle-aged males (Marmot et al., 2006: 116).

Work is not exclusively the domain of paid employment. Work in the home, and the division of this labor between genders, interacts with labor market pressures to affect health. This creates an important additional dimension when considering the relationship between work and health, especially for women, who bear most of the domestic responsibility. A study in Spain found that female workers who were married (or living as a couple) had poorer health than males. Further, family demands had a greater negative impact on the health of female manual workers than for female non-manual workers. The authors argue that the division of nonpaid work must be considered in conjunction with paid employment in any explanation of health (Artazcoz, Borrell, and Benach, 2001).

The implications of both demand–control and effort–reward are roughly the same. Poor health results are linked to frustration and lack of control in the work environment, and these are found much more often at the lower ends of the job hierarchy than they are higher up.

The new productivity-enhancing techniques, and workers' concerted action to claim their share of the gains, led to improved living conditions and much reduced the incidence of infectious disease and early childhood death, but they also contributed to a lack of control and reward because of changes in the labor process. It may be difficult to believe given the organization of work today, but in the beginning of the industrial age, craft workers exercised control over the work process: tools, work time, intensity, product quality, and conditions of work were under the subjective control of those who did the work, at least among skilled craft workers. By the early twentieth century, however, "scientific management" pioneered by US engineer Frederick Taylor aimed not just to increase productivity, but also to deliberately wrest control of the labor process from workers and place it in the hands of management. Work was broken into small, discrete parts, each of which was timed to maximize the intensity of workers' efforts. The conditions of labor, instruments of labor, and the product of labor were all determined by management and kept out of labor's control (Braverman, 1974).

The diversity and interest of work known to the craft worker gave way to the increasingly repetitive and simplified movements of the factory process, as changing techniques—exemplified by the assembly line—required a decreasing use of the varied muscular and mental abilities of the laborer. Work became increasingly stultifying and debilitating as it was forced to obey the demands of machinery. In contrast with the craft worker, the factory worker loses the varied use of muscles: both the intellectual and physical creativity of the work process are dramatically reduced. In the hands of capital, the machine does not free labor from work, but deprives the work of useful exercise and interest. The self-regulating pace and rest of work known to the skilled craft worker was transformed into the externally determined conditions of labor imposed on increasingly semi-skilled and unskilled factory workers. All of this affected workers' health. As a recent indicator of how this negatively impacts health results, between 1997 and 2001 professionals in England and Wales lived an average of 8.4 years longer than manual workers. Further, the number of health-related problems is higher for manual workers, and these unequal results persist even when the differences in behavior of the two groups (professionals eat better—again begging the question why this is the case) are taken into consideration (Cutler, Deacon, and Lleras-Muney, 2006: 99).

Unemployment and insecurity

Unemployment has been linked to increased mortality, worse mental health, and unhealthy behavioral changes such as alcohol consumption and marriage breakdown. In terms of stressful life events, unemployment is ranked as equivalent to the death of a family member. Interestingly, the stress is still present even when the income consequences of unemployment are not as severe, as would be the case if unemployment benefits were particularly generous. Both men and women who are unemployed report being in bad health more often than those who are employed (McKee-Ryan et al., 2005; Bartley, Ferrie, and Montgomery, 2006: 85). When unemployment does lead to financial strain, as has been the case in the United States, which has very limited unemployment insurance programs compared with other developed nations, it has an even larger negative impact. People who become unemployed and have to borrow money are more likely to suffer from depression, and report poorer health than unemployed people who do not have to borrow (White, 1991). A study of European nations found that although all unemployed people reported worse health conditions than the employed, the inequality was worse in countries that had less generous means-tested unemployment benefits (as is the case in the United States) (Bambra and Eikemo, 2008).

Since unemployment in the United States has been relatively low between 1995 and 2008, we might expect the negative health impacts associated with joblessness to be on the decline. Yet this is not necessarily the case. People do not have to be faced with the dreaded layoff notice to suffer from the trauma associated with unemployment. Poor-quality, temporary jobs in environments with little financial protection for the unemployed can create economic insecurity even for those with work. One study looking at the health status of British civil servants facing privatization found that people's health became worse, including cardiovascular risk factors, during the period of uncertainty and instability just before the announcement (Ferrie et al., 1995). A European study found that stress from lack of control is greater among non-permanent employees than for permanent workers (Gimeno et al., 2004). Recent research has linked obesity to economic insecurity. Obesity is one-third higher in countries like the United States and Canada than it is in countries like Norway and Sweden. The weight difference is not because of Scandinavians' greater love of sport, or the increased availability of fast food in the United States. Rather, the authors found that it is the stress of life in an economic environment without a social safety net that contributes to obesity in the Anglo nations (Offer, Pechey, and Ulijaszek, 2010). Having precarious employment may not be much of a health advantage over having no employment.

Studies relating work to health impacts are quite controversial because it is very difficult to determine in which direction the causation runs. Does health deteriorate because of work, or do people who are less healthy have worse jobs and more frequent unemployment? It certainly seems possible that, in a flexible labor market, people who took more sick days and exhibited worse health would be the among the first to be let go, and so it is entirely possible that poor health increases the chance of unemployment. Yet this does not mean that causation does not run the other way. According to the authors of one survey on the subject, "The evidence of health effects arising from unemployment is sufficiently substantial to consider the relationship causal" (Mustard, Lavis, and Ostry, 2006: 177). A more nuanced approach is to acknowledge that work (or lack of work) and poor health interact and accumulate over a lifetime (Bartley et al., 2006: 88).

The impact of unemployment is different now than it was during the early industrial stage of capitalism, in which lack of support for the unemployed and the precarious incomes of the working class resulted in genuine penury for the out of work, making them susceptible to infectious disease. Yet the current impacts of unemployment are debilitating nonetheless. It results in considerable financial and emotional stress, which leads to quantifiably worse health results and behaviors. Further, it is not only the actual pink slip that gives rise to health problems, but increased instability while still at work. It follows that policies that create full employment and stable, secure jobs should lead to superior health outcomes.

Occupational illness

It is one of the greatest achievements of our society that the once satanic mills are no longer as hellish, at least in the developed world where greater workplace safety has been won over generations of hard struggle. Working conditions are no longer as obviously debilitating as the horrors described in Chapter 3. Yet, despite these gains, US workers should be under no illusions that their places of employment are safe. According to the International Labour Organization, in the United States an average of more than 6,000 workers a year died in work fatalities in the decade between 1992 and 2002 (ILO, 2009). An international comparison of accident rates is a crude measure because countries have different industrial structures with different occupational risks (for example Canada has a relatively high proportion of employment in the dangerous mining and resources sector). However the US accident rate of 4.9 per 100,000 workers in 2001 is above the 3.5 average of the EU12 and well above the 1.5 rate of Sweden (ILO, 2005). This statistic only documents sudden violent deaths, like a mine collapse. Workers also die in much slower, more insidious ways, such as black lung disease or exposure to asbestos. To illustrate the prevalence of this problem, one study found that in 1992 more than 60,000 disease fatalities could be traced to occupational causes. When injuries and illnesses were combined, the total cost in 1992 was estimated at $171 billion (Leigh et al., 1997).

The problems of chronic occupational disease have been recognized for decades, even by industry itself, although as with environmental connections to illness, the specific links and mechanisms are difficult to pinpoint. In 1978, the US National Institute of Occupational Safety and Health (NIOSH) estimated that 20 to 40 percent of all cancers were occupational in origin. Outraged, the American Industrial Health Council, an industry-funded organization, hired its own expert, Dr. R. Stallones, to refute this finding. But it couldn't be done. Instead, he concluded that 20 percent of all cancers were work-related. Specific links between blue-collar work and elevated cancer have been found in the steel, auto, mining, aluminum, rubber, carbon electrode, pesticide use and production, petroleum, and cobalt metal industries (Katz, 2012: 100). It is not only the more industrial occupations that are hazardous to health. Dry cleaners have elevated rates of digestive tract cancers, and the IARC ranks hairdressing as probably carcinogenic (Chernomas and Hudson, 2007: 126).

Many of the health problems identified in the environmental section are occupational problems as well. Workers producing dyes, solvents, paints, and other petroleum products are at greater risk of cancer. For example, trichloroethylene has been linked with cancers of the esophagus, liver, and kidney as well as non-Hodgkins lymphoma (Irigaray et al., 2007: 649). Agriculture is also a dangerous occupation. Compared with the rest of society, farmers have a higher rate of mortality from several forms of cancer. Migrant farm laborers have a higher than average incidence of testis, stomach, and prostate cancers (Clapp et al., 2007: 637). A list of some occupational hazards can be found in Table 4.1 (overleaf). All of this information casts considerable doubt on the ACS estimate that occupational exposure counts for about 4 percent of cancers in the United States (ACS, 2010: 50).

So while cholesterol, smoking, high blood pressure, toxic air and water are clearly some of the factors in mortality for heart disease and cancer, by themselves they cannot account for the differences in social patterns of diseases. The conditions of employment are also important factors. Work at the lower ends of the occupational hierarchy, with less control and fewer rewards, creates health problems. Further, unemployment and insecure jobs create stress. Finally, many jobs can be hazardous to people's short and long-term health. It follows that a political economy that exacerbates these conditions, creating more unstable jobs with less control in dangerous conditions, will create more health problems.

INEQUALITY

Beyond the specifics of the labor process, inequality and social position have important health determinants, even in a wealthy society. Figure 4.2 shows the connection between life expectancy and an index of socio-economic well-being made up of income, education, poverty rates, unemployment, and job skills. In the United States there is a pronounced gradient, where those in more deprived groups have a lower life expectancy than those in richer groups. Further, this inequality has widened between the early 1980s and the late 1990s (Singh and Siahpush, 2006). Wealthier people have a lower incidence of high blood pressure and of cholesterol, and tend to live longer. This result is amazingly consistent across nations. In a 2008 study of 16 developed nations, every one showed that mortality decreased with income for both men and women. This result held for virtually all causes of death. Most of the illnesses responsible for the decreases in longevity of the poor were not correctable with health interventions, placing the emphasis clearly on societal conditions rather than revising the medical system (Berkman and Epstein, 2008: 2509). People in the bottom 5 percent

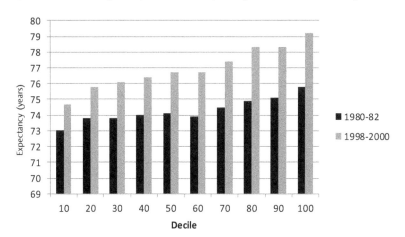

Figure 4.2 Relationship between neighborhood socio-economic decile and life expectancy at birth in the United States, 1980–82 and 1998–2000

Source: Singh and Siahpush (2006).

Table 4.1 Dangers associated with workplace exposure to high-volume carcinogens

Chemical	Sites of primary cancer [a,b,c]	Other chronic health effects [d,e]
Acrylonitrile	Colon, lung	Eye and nose irritant, gastrointestinal effects, jaundice, mild anemia
Arsenic	Skin, lung, liver, lymphatic system	Gastrointestinal disturbances, hyperpigmentation, peripheral neuropathy, hemolytic anemia, dermatitis, bronchitis, nasal system ulceration
Asbestos	Lung, plural and peritoneal mesothelioma, gastrointestinal tract	Asbestosis (pulmonary fibrosis, pleural plaques, and pleural calcification), anorexia, weight loss
Beryllium	Lung	Dermatitis, bronchitis, respiratory effects
Benzene	Bone marrow (leukemia)	Central nervous system and gastrointestinal effects, blood abnormalities (anemia, leukopenia, and thrombocytopenia)
Cadmium	Prostate, respiratory tract, renal	Renal disease, respiratory effects
Carbon tetrachloride	Liver	Cirrhosis and liver disease, kidney and gastrointestinal effects, dermatitis, jaundice
Chromium	Nasal cavity and sinuses, lung, larynx	Dermatitis, skin ulceration, nasal system ulceration, bronchitis, bronchopneumonia, inflammation of the larynx and liver
Ethylene oxide	Leukemia, gastric cancer (suggested)	Mutagenic, respiratory irritant
Nickel	Nasal cavity and sinuses, lung	Dermatitis
Vinyl chloride	Angioscarcoma-lung, brain, haemato-lymphopoietic	Reproductive and central nervous system, Reynaud's syndrome, acroosteolysis

Primary sources: [a] Davis and Rall (1981); [b] Cole and Goldman (1975); [c] U.S Department of Health and Education, and Welfare (1977); [d] Casarett and Doull (1975); [e] Waldbott (1978); [f] International Agency of Research on Cancer (1979); [g] National Institute for Occupational Safety and Health (1981).
Source: Davis (2007, Table 10-1, p. 258).

Occupations at risk[b]	Latency period for cancer (years)[b,f]	Risk ratios for cancer[b,f]	1981 NIOSH estimated no. of workers exposed[g]	
			Full+ part time	Full time
Chemical workers and plastic workers	20+	4–6	374,345	55,706
Miners, smelters, insecticide makers and sprayers, chemical workers, oil refiners, vintners	10+	3–8	255,277 432,017 (arsenic oxides)	5,926 596
Miners, millers, textile, insulation and shipyard workers	4–40	1.5–12	1,280,202	449,960
Beryllium workers, defense and aerospace industry, nuclear industry	15+	1,5–2	855,189	632
Explosives, benzene and rubber cement workers, distillers, dye users, printers, shoemakers	6–14	2–3	1,495,706	147,604
Electrical workers, painters, battery plant and alloy workers		2.5	1,376,871	38,433
Dry-cleaning machinists			1,380,232	64,023
Producers, processors and users of Cr: acetylene and aniline workers; bleachers, glass pottery, and linoleum workers; battery makers	5–15	3–4	1,451,631 (oxides)	59,946
Hospital workers, laboratory workers, fumigators			144,152	107,455
Nickel smelters, mixers and roasters, electrolysis workers	3–30	5–10 (lung) 100+ (nasal, sinuses)	1,369,278 (oxides)	51,840
Plastic industry	20+		239,375	29,838

of the income distribution in 1980 had a life expectancy at all ages that was about 25 percent lower than the corresponding life expectancies of those in the top 5 percent of the income distribution (Rogot et al., 1992).

A study examining health indicators, such as mortality, health status, and activity limitation, of both children and adults found a clear health gradient between the wealthiest, middle, and lowest income groups (Braverman et al., 2010). In the United States, the risk of stroke is 80 percent lower for those with some university education than those without a high school diploma. The incidence of diabetes is two times higher in people who have not completed high school compared with those with a BA. Once people reach 25, college graduates live five years longer than those who do not finish high school. If every person in the United States were to have the mortality rate of those who attended (even if they did not graduate from) university, it would save seven times as many lives as all biomedical advances (Woolf, 2011: 1902). The incidence of cardiac arrest in the poorest 25 percent of neighborhoods in four big US cities is almost double that in the richest quartile (Reinier et al., 2011).

In the United Kingdom, people in the poorest neighborhoods die, on average, seven years earlier than those from the wealthiest. They are also sick for much longer while they are alive. The difference between richest and poorest in disability-free life expectancy is 17 years. The gradient between rich and poor holds for all ranks in society, not just the extreme high and low ends (Marmot, 2010: 16). As Harvey Brenner confidently declared, "It is now among the firmest of epidemiological findings ... higher income has been routinely shown to be a significant inverse predictor of morbidity and mortality" (2005: 1,215). The question is not whether or not there are social inequalities in health: poor people tend to die younger in virtually all societies, and it is a matter of the systemic reasons why this occurs.

Those with a higher socio-economic status tend to smoke less, eat healthier foods, and generally have healthier lifestyles. These inequalities can have intergenerational effects since parents' income has an important impact on their children's diets, which in turn influence adult health (Dubois, 2006: 148). In the United Kingdom, between 1994 and 1996 only 19 percent of 2 to 5-year-olds below the poverty line consumed a "good diet," compared with a still dismal, but considerably better, 28 percent of those above the poverty line (Dubois, 2006: 154). We have suggested

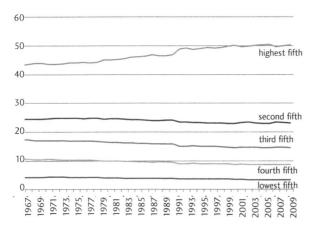

Figure 4.3 Percentage of total income earned by quintile, United States, 1967 to 2007

Source: US Census Bureau, Current Population Survey, Annual Social and Economic Supplements.

that these choices are heavily influenced by people's place in the socio-economic hierarchy. According to Michael Marmot, "social inequalities in health arise because of inequalities in the conditions of daily life and the fundamental drivers that give rise to them: inequities in power, money and resources" (2010: 16).

Between 1930 and 1980, the United States, and other developed nations, put in place wide-ranging policies aimed at reducing disparity. Progressive income taxes, welfare, favorable rules for unions, and minimum wages are all examples of a broad attempt to reduce the gap between rich and poor. These policies were successful. US income distribution in this period became more equal and the percentage of poor people decreased. In the decade between 1960 and 1970 the percentage of people below the poverty level dropped from 18 percent to 8 percent (Navarro, 1984: 522). After 1980, for reasons explained below, these policies were reversed, with predictable consequences. Between 1967 and 2009, the share of total income that was earned by the wealthiest 20 percent of the population has increased from 44 percent to 50 percent. Figure 4.3 shows that the other 80 percent of the population have actually taken home a lower share of income. The real gains have come at the very top of the income spectrum. In fact, the higher up the income spectrum, the larger the gains during this period. The top 5 percent of earners saw their share of income increase from 17 to 22 percent. According to inequality experts Thomas Piketty and Emmanuel

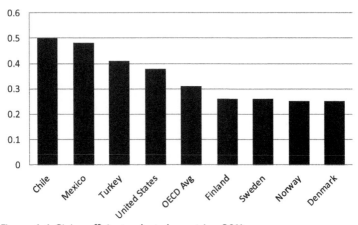

Figure 4.4 Gini coefficient, selected countries, 2011

Source: OECD (2011).

Saez, between 1973 and 2000 the average income of the bottom 90 percent of US taxpayers fell by 7 percent. Incomes of the top 1 percent rose by 148 percent, the top 0.1 percent by 343 percent, and for the extremely well off in the top 0.01 percent they rose by an amazing 599 percent (Piketty and Saez, 2003). The United States is also one of the most unequal developed nations. The Gini coefficient is a measure of income inequality on a scale from zero to one. A coefficient of 1 would indicate that one extremely rich person earned all of the income in a nation. Figure 4.4 shows the Gini coefficient in the United States was 0.38, surpassed in inequality by only Mexico, Turkey, and Chile. The OECD average was 0.31 and the Scandinavian countries had a much greater degree of equality, with coefficients around 0.25.

Although rich people have better health outcomes than poor people, income equality in a society improves health. Income inequality is strongly associated with a variety of adverse health measures such as age-adjusted death rates, low birth weight, crime rates, and incarceration rates (Poland et al., 1998: 790). In the tribute to equality, the 2009 book *The Spirit Level*, one of the many scores on which more equal societies outperform less equal ones is on health. In the United States, people live four years longer in more equal states. Internationally, looking at 23 wealthy countries, infant mortality is lowest among countries that have the lowest income inequality (see Figure 4.5) (Navarro et al., 2003; Wilkinson and Pickett, 2009). A study attempting to explain the improved health performance of Canada relative to the United States over the last 50

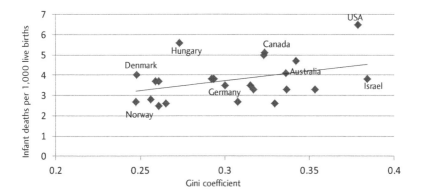

Figure 4.5 Income inequality and infant mortality in 23 developed nations

Source: OECD, Infant mortality deaths per 1000 and Gini coefficients of income inequality (www.oecd.org/statistics/).

years concluded that Canada's greater income equality (and public healthcare provision) were the two dominant factors (Hertzman and Siddiqi, 2008).

Historically, people live longer in countries where income inequality is the smallest. The loss of common purpose, perceptions of unfairness, disrespect, and lack of trust that evolve from inequality of income may in turn result in inequalities in health outcomes. Even health results that are seemingly the result of lifestyle choices are heavily influenced by the broader economic context in which people live.

Black and white? Race and class

Readers familiar with US research on inequality and health will no doubt be wondering at the dearth of comment on race. Official data sources certainly lean in the opposite direction. Unlike most other wealthy nations, the United States does not routinely report health statistics by class, but does so by race (Kawachi, Daniels, and Robinson, 2005: 343). This is not to suggest that race is unimportant, although it is "of limited biological significance" (Williams, Lavizzo-Mourey, and Warren, 1994: 26). However, race does impact on health because of how it interrelates with class to form "codeterminants" of health (Kawachi et al., 2005). If we were forced to choose between race and class as competing explanations of health, class would at first glance be the obvious choice. Once socio-economic class is accounted for, there is little difference between blacks and whites. In terms of health, low-income blacks have much more in common with low-income whites than with more affluent blacks (Kawachi et al., 2005).

Yet to declare that therefore race is unimportant would be a gross oversimplification for two reasons. First, even within socio-economic classes, there are different health outcomes. For example, at similar levels of family income, blacks have a higher rate of heart disease than whites. Second, race influences class position. It is therefore not sufficient to point out that low-income people have similar health outcomes (and worse outcomes than richer people) without also acknowledging that blacks are more likely to be poor than whites. In 2010, 27 percent of US blacks were poor (defined as having income below a certain threshold—for a family of two adults and two children it was $22,000) compared with 10 percent of non-Hispanic whites (National Poverty Center, 2010). As a result of the impact of race on socio-economic class, minorities will be over-represented in the negative social and environmental conditions associated with poverty. Louisiana's "Cancer Alley" is not only poor, it is also home to a much larger minority population than the national average. In Massachusetts, communities with larger minority populations were more likely to contain environmental hazards. Communities with a minority population of over 25 percent had on average 27 environmental hazards, compared with an average of only three hazards for communities with in which minorities made up less than 5 percent of the population (Faber and Krieg 2002; see also Ash et al., 2009).

So race is an important factor in explaining health outcomes, but just not in as straightforward a manner as it is often presented. Race matters because class matters, and race influences what class people end up in.

Public health is improved when food is safer, the workplace contains fewer hazards, and the environment in which we live contains fewer pollutants. Health results are much worse for those at the lower ends of both the workplace and income hierarchy. Finally, for high-income countries, higher levels of inequality are associated with poorer health results. Given these facts, it is little surprise that the United States ranks poorly in health outcomes. Beginning in the late 1970s, the political and economic structure in the United States was dramatically transformed in response to falling corporate profitability in a manner that worsened every one of these factors.

THE RECENT US POLITICAL ECONOMY:
A TURN FOR THE WORSE

The late 1970s were a traumatic period for the United States. On the economic front there was a great deal of hand wringing about the nation's declining dominance. It is certainly true that the profitability of US firms had slipped considerably since its high water mark after the Second World War (Duménil and Lévy, 2002). Even among economists who focus on profits as the key determinant of economic success, the cause of the decline is a matter of considerable controversy (Gordon, Bowles, and Weisskopf, 1994; Duménil and Lévy, 2002; Brenner, 2006; Shaikh, 2011). What is less controversial is that, under the banner of neoliberalism, the corporate world started a highly successful campaign to change the political and economic structure of the United States in order to correct for what it claimed were the main drags on profits. These wide-ranging changes involved reducing regulations that increased costs to firms, privatization, and making the labor market more hostile to workers. The evidence presented in the previous section suggests that political and economic conditions have a strong influence on chronic disease. Public health will become worse when the quality of the food we eat becomes less nourishing, the environment in which we live more hazardous, the conditions of work more unstable, and society more unequal. Unfortunately, this is exactly what has happened in the United States over the last 30 years.

Regulation

One of the explanations for the struggles of the US economy in the late 1970s was that it was over-regulated. It was true that government in the United States had expanded legislation that limited the harmful actions of firms after the Second World War. The most visible embodiment of this trend was perhaps the creation of the EPA in 1970 and the Occupational Safety and Health Administration (OSHA) in 1971. The pressure for the OSHA came largely from the union movement, and was a reflection of its historically relatively strong position after the Second World War (discussed in the next section). The EPA, and the regulations that it oversaw, were the result of broader coalitions. The rise of environmental regulations is worth a closer look because there are some important parallels with the movement to enhance public health after 1900 discussed in the previous chapter. Infectious disease was partly conquered by government intervention to create a healthier urban environment through things such as sanitation and regulations to ensure food quality. Environmental regulations were, in part, an attempt by a broad coalition of groups in society to alleviate the negative health impacts of pollution.

The origins of the modern environmental movement are commonly traced to the publication of several books that alerted the public to the growing danger of chemical pollutants, the most prominent of which was Rachel Carson's *Silent Spring* in 1962. Polling data during the 1960s showed that environmental issues gripped the US public with an "unprecedented speed and urgency" (Kraft, 2011: 97). The environmental movement comprised those concerned with a wide range of interrelated issues, including wilderness conservation, resource depletion, pollution control, and of course public health. It was a part of, and borrowed tactics from, the broader social movements in the 1960s. It also illustrated the increasing willingness of these groups to seek political solutions that constrained the profit-seeking activities of businesses when they were deemed harmful to society. The first half of the 1970s was the most active period for legislated environmental protection in US history. Regulations were passed on air pollution, water pollution, regulation of pesticides, ocean conservation, and control of toxic substances (Kraft, 2011: 95). At the time, it appeared as though broad public mobilization had pressured the government into passing radical legislation to protect people and their environment from some of the worst damage caused by private business.

Yet, as the example of the Clean Air Act (CAA) demonstrates, the main theme in US environmental policy is that in the conflict between public groups and corporate interests, it is corporate interests that tend to win the day. This is not to say that business has a completely free hand. The dramatic strengthening of the CAA in 1970 was, like the other environmental regulations, a response to concerns about the environment, but it was also about the negative health impacts of poor air quality in many cities. Yet the post-1970 record of the CAA is one of regulatory weakness and business influence. Of the several hundreds of airborne pollutants, the EPA only managed to set limits on seven between 1970 and 1990 (Gonzalez, 2001: 95).

When the CAA was amended in 1990 to encompass 189 substances, the process was heavily influenced by the business lobby. Pressure to broaden the CAA came from environmental organizations, church groups, unions such as the US Steelworkers, and public health advocates such as the US Lung Association, organized into the National Clean Air Coalition (NCAC). However, the business community, especially automobile manufacturers, also wanted the federal government to step in and harmonize the patchwork of clean air legislation that had developed in different states in response to the lack of action taken at a national level since 1970. In the battle over what form the 1990 CAA would take, the business community organized under the banner of the Clean Air Working Group (CAWG), dominated by the auto, oil, and chemical industries (Gonzalez, 2001: 102). CAWG served the dual function of being the lead organization in lobbying for a version of the CAA favorable to firms and acting as an arena to coordinate a consensus within the business community. CAWG worked through the 1980s to develop policies that it would like to see implemented on twelve separate clean air issues, and was sufficiently influential in the policy-formulation process that even the chemical and oil industry could support the 1990 CAA. In contrast, the NCAC was largely excluded from the policy-making process (Gonzalez, 2001: 111).

As was the case with the CAA, US environmental regulation more generally can best be described as a symbolic, technical fix to allay public concerns (Gonzalez, 2005: 9). During the formation of the EPA and passage of the CAA, popular pressure for increased regulation forced business to exchange some regulatory oversight for stability. Yet the regulations were constrained by the "primacy of capitalist imperatives," in that they did not compromise profitability more than was absolutely necessary to alleviate the public pressure (Gonzalez, 2005: 21). Similarly, when automobile pollution became a public health issue in California, the regulatory solution was limited to the technological fix of environmental modernization of cars, using innovations such as the catalytic converter. More sweeping regulatory changes that would have broader implications on the profits of car companies and real estate developers, such as reducing the number of cars on the road or limiting urban sprawl, were never seriously considered (Gonzalez, 2005: 87).

Even when business is influential in policy formulation, as was the case with the CAA, the costs of regulation can be very high. Protective regulation such as the CAA's increases costs to firms in a number of ways, making them less competitive in the more global economy. The most obvious was the compliance cost of meeting government rules, but the tax revenue required to fund the monitoring and enforcement arms needed to give the regulations actual muscle also came in part from the corporate world. According to the EPA the compliance costs of the CAA were around $50 billion in 2010. However, the CAA illustrates that the advantages of regulation can often exceed the costs.

In spite of business influence the CAA has achieved some important successes. Between 1970 and 1979, sulfur dioxide and carbon monoxide in the air decreased by 40 percent. Suspended particulate matter declined by 17 percent (Navarro, 1984: 523). Between 1990 and 2008 carbon monoxide levels fell by 68 percent and sulfur dioxide by 59 percent. Toxic pollutant emissions dropped by 40 percent between 1990 and 2005 (EPA, 2010: 1). Although not all of these reductions can be attributed directly to the CAA—some might be due to a change in industrial structure in the United States, for example—the Act was directly responsible for an estimated $1.3 trillion in 2010 in decreased mortality and improved environmental conditions (EPA, 2011: 2). The $50 billion cost to business pales in comparison with over $1 trillion in benefits to the nation, suggesting that many other environmental improvements might be worthwhile on efficiency grounds alone. It is important to remember that many other countries impose these kinds of regulatory costs on their businesses to protect the interests of their citizenry.

These gains would not have been achieved without the mobilization of the broad coalition of groups that pressured the US government to pass the various versions of the CAA, but the legislation was also limited and structured heavily by the power of business in the political process. Even when regulatory benefits exceed its costs, different groups in society tend to bear the costs and reap the benefits unevenly. In the kind of protective legislation being discussed in this section, the cost is borne primarily by the affected firms (or maybe their customers if they are in a position to pass on the cost of the regulation). The benefits are felt by either the workers, in the case of the OSHA, or society at large in the case of the EPA. Even regulation for which the benefits exceed the costs for society as a whole will often be opposed by the business community because its expenses will increase. The majority of people actually favored strengthening regulations like the EPA's CAA in the early 1980s, but these programs were cut because of the adamant refusal of business to take financial responsibility for its own pollution (Navarro, 1984: 523).

Declining funding

The post-1980 history of all three protective regulatory agencies (OSHA, EPA, and the Food and Drug Administration, FDA) is remarkably similar. A number of crafty methods were developed to shackle them without taking the drastic, and perhaps politically dangerous, step of eliminating the entire organizations. Agencies were populated with political appointees, especially during the Republican years, which usually resulted in a head ideologically opposed to the very mandate of the particular organization. Agency budgets were slashed, limiting their ability to monitor and enforce their regulatory mandate. Between 1981 and 1984, the budgets of regulatory agencies in the United States fell by 11 percent overall. The EPA's budget fell by 35 percent. The staff of the EPA was reduced from 14,075 to 10,392 (Blyth, 2002: 181–5). Referrals by the EPA to the Justice Department for the prosecution of violators fell by 84 percent, and the number of enforcement orders fell by 33 percent. The FDA budget was cut by 30 percent over this period, and its enforcement orders declined by 88 percent. "Between 1981 and 1984, the absolute number of regulations in the Federal Register declined by 25 percent, and since 1984, no new permanent regulatory department has been authorized or established by the federal government" (Blyth, 2002: 181–5).

The budget-cutting trends of the early 1980s have not changed. With its limited staffing levels, state-run OSHA enforcement could, on average, only inspect each workplace once every 55 years. The average federal fine for a "serious" violation in 1995 was $763, and the maximum fine was only around $7,000 (Weil, 1996; McQuiston, Ronda, and Loomis, 1998). The EPA's Office of Prevention, Pesticides, and Toxic Substances had its staff cut from 600 to 320 in 2009 (Reuben, 2010: 19). The EPA is supposed to monitor chemicals under the Toxic Substances Control Act (TSCA), but it does not require companies to perform toxicity tests (in fact, it discourages them because if the tests are positive the company must report it). The EPA has required the testing of only 1 percent of commercial chemicals currently available, has regulated only five and has not attempted to ban one since 1991 (Reuben, 2010: 22). After inflation, its budget fell by 25 percent between 2004 and 2009 (Union of Concerned Scientists, 2008: 19). A 2006 subcommittee reviewing the FDA Science Board concluded that the agency was "not prepared to meet regulatory responsibilities," in part because after inflation its budget was $300 million less in 2007 than it was in 2008 (Reuben, 2010: 19).

Trade agreements as a social determinant of health

Regulation that increases costs to firms is difficult to maintain in a free trade area because profit-maximizing companies tend to produce

David Graham versus Vioxx

Dr. David Graham is the associate director for science and medicine in the FDA Office of Drug Safety. His medical, epidemiological, and biostatistics training was received from Johns Hopkins, Yale, and the University of Pennsylvania. Despite this rigorous training, his ability as a researcher was called into question when he blew the whistle on Vioxx, a drug that has caused some 100,000 heart attacks and 50,000 deaths in the United States.

According to Graham, the FDA "reacted violently" when he announced he was going to submit his research for peer review. His supervisors described his work as "scientific rumor," and his director called the study "junk science." The day after his supervisor's remarks, Graham's study was the lead article in the *Journal of the American Medical Association*, which was accompanied by a call for a complete restructuring of the FDA. After Graham's study was published, the FDA contacted a key senator and accused Graham of being a "liar, cheat, bully, a demagogue and untrustworthy." It contacted the Government Accountability Project with the same line of character assassination. Graham's director contacted the editor of the *Lancet* and accused him of scientific misconduct, the highest crime a scientist can commit.

According to Graham, the FDA's angry response was a result of its willingness to sacrifice safety for its own revenue. In 2002, the FDA collected fees from the pharmaceutical industry, under the Prescription Drug User Fee Act, of $143.3 million, most of the $209.8 million total operating costs for reviewing drugs. Graham went on to argue that the FDA approach is to virtually disregard safety as something to be managed "in the post-marketing setting," the effect of which is that "our parents, and grandparents, our children get to be the guinea pigs in the grand experiment while drug companies continue to make profits." Graham's policy prescription is that industry cannot be the client. Public health must be funded by the public, via an institution run by and for the public.

If we do not wish to be the guinea pigs, a proper study on drugs like Vioxx should take longer and be much larger than those that serve industry interests. "If you are making $3 billion a year selling a drug, every day of clinical trials is another day you are not making $10 million" (Graham, 2004: 25). Two-thirds of FDA scientists are not confident that products approved by the FDA are safe. Eighteen say they have been pressured to change their own conclusions.

in the lowest-cost jurisdiction. In addition, free trade agreements made in the neoliberal period reflected a pro-business policy bias by including specific provisions that deterred governments from strengthening protective legislation that could potentially harm firms. For example, the World Trade Organization (WTO) dispute resolution tribunal ruled that the European Union's ban on beef from cattle treated with artificial hormones violated the principle of free trade after the United States lodged a complaint. The EU ban was based on the precautionary principle (we return to this in Chapter 6), under which substances must be proven safe before they are sold. The WTO ruled that the precautionary principle imposed too heavy a burden of proof on the producer, and allowed the United States to take retaliatory action against the European Union (Shaffer and Brenner, 2004: 82).

Another highly controversial example of trade rules that could potentially have negative health impacts is Chapter Eleven of the North American Free Trade Agreement (NAFTA), between Canada, the United States, and Mexico. It was intended to protect foreign investors from having their property arbitrarily seized by governments, but its wording creates scope for any foreign business that is harmed by legislative changes to sue the offending government (Dougherty, 2007).

NAFTA tribunals have not been very consistent in applying this rule. The Ethyl Corporation, a US manufacturer of a gasoline additive (MMT), sued the Canadian government in 1996 after it banned MMT because of its links to cancer. As part of the 1998 settlement, the Government of Canada removed the ban, was forced to issue a statement that there was no evidence of harm caused by the product, and paid the company approximately $20 million (Canadian). MMT is banned in many US states and in Europe (Canadian Centre for Policy Alternatives, 1998). Conversely, a Canadian company, Methanex, is the world's largest producer of methanol, the key ingredient in the gasoline additive MTBE (methyl tertiary butyl ether). In 1995, MTBE began to turn up in wells throughout California, and by 1999 had contaminated 30 public water systems. The state ordered that the additive be phased out, after some research linked it to cancer and other human health problems. Methanex filed suit under NAFTA's Chapter Eleven, seeking $970 million in compensation for loss of market share and consequently future profits. A 2005 NAFTA tribunal ruled against Methanex's claim of expropriation (Waitzkin, 2011: 76). The two contrasting results demonstrate the uncertainty surrounding Chapter

Eleven. It is still possible for governments to enact protective legislation, even if it constrains the profitability of firms, without being found liable under Chapter Eleven. However, the possibility of a successful suit, like that of the Ethyl Corporation remains a very real possibility given the wording of Chapter Eleven. At the very least governments must now be concerned with defending themselves against companies that consider themselves harmed by what, before the introduction of Chapter Eleven, would have been straightforward decisions on health and environmental policy.

Industry influence on regulations

Businesses have become so active in influencing the activities of regulatory agencies that one author argues that it is the "modus operandi of at least a large proportion of corporations in the United States" (Bohme, Zorabedian, and Egilman, 2005: 338). For their part, the regulatory agencies have often been willing participants in their own emasculation. OSHA currently works in very close collaboration with industry. An agreement between the agency and the industry trade association, the American Chemistry Council (ACC), states that one of its goals is to "provide expertise in the development of training and education program for [OSHA's] Voluntary Protection Program evaluators and Responsible Care auditors" (Davis, 2007: 386). A study examining the nutrition-related health problems in the United States found that the "food industry seems to exert a big influence on the development of food policies" (Dubois, 2006: 138). Another study on regulation of chemicals found that "as a result of regulatory weaknesses and a powerful lobby, the chemicals industry operates virtually unfettered by regulation or accountability for harm its products may cause" (Reuben, 2010: 23). Regulatory agencies facing budgetary constraints, under political pressure not to impose costs on business, and facing a powerful industry lobby have become shells of their former protective selves.

Firms lobbied politicians to change the regulatory rules—as when the Department of Labor under President George W. Bush changed the way toxins were measured in the workplace, making it more difficult for the OSHA to find them harmful to workers (Leonnig, 2008: A01). They also used the courts: a court challenge from industry forced OSHA to scrap a 1979 ruling that set the standard for benzene, a known carcinogen, at one part per million (ppm), rolling the requirements back to the earlier 10 ppm requirement. This was despite 1989 and 2005 studies that found that Chinese

FDA and BPA

Bisphenol A (BPA), an important component of water bottles and infant formula containers, has been linked with testicular cancer, breast cancer, and diabetes, and was suspected to be harmful to children's development even in low doses. Despite hundreds of studies showing that it was harmful to animals in low doses, the FDA announced in 2008 that it was safe on the basis of two studies funded by the Society of the Plastics Industry. One of the studies was never subject to peer review and never published, and the other suffered from important methodological shortcomings (Rust, 2008). The balance of scientific evidence forced the FDA to modify its stance slightly by 2010, stating that although low levels of exposure were safe, "recent studies using novel approaches to test for subtle effects" had created some concern about the impacts of BPA on fetuses, children and infants (US Department of Health and Human Services, 2010).

By 2010 many countries, including Canada, had banned the use of BPA in products aimed at infants, but the FDA was bound by a law that prevented it from banning its use in products for which there are no substitutes. On its website the FDA lamented the limits to its regulatory reach:

> Current BPA food contact uses were approved under food additive regulations issued more than 40 years ago. This regulatory structure limits the oversight and flexibility of FDA.
>
> Once a food additive is approved, any manufacturer of food or food packaging may use the food additive in accordance with the regulation. There is no requirement to notify FDA of that use.
>
> For example, today there exist hundreds of different formulations for BPA-containing epoxy linings, which have varying characteristics. As currently regulated, manufacturers are not required to disclose to FDA the existence or nature of these formulations.
>
> Furthermore, if FDA were to decide to revoke one or more approved uses, FDA would need to undertake what could be a lengthy process of rulemaking to accomplish this goal.
>
> (US Department of Health and Human Services, 2010)

workers exposed to benzene were statistically more likely to develop cancers of bone marrow, lung cancer, and leukemia, even those with exposure levels between "6 to 10 ppm" (Davis, 2007: 384–6).

Industry also influenced enforcement and penalties. For example, 42 percent of EPA scientists knew of instances where "commercial interests have inappropriately induced the reversal or withdrawal of EPA scientific conclusions or decisions through political intervention" (Union of Concerned Scientists, 2008: 23). In response to industry pressure, the National Toxicology Program (NTP) delayed listing fiberglass insulation for nearly six years, and removed saccharin from its Report on Carcinogens (RoC) (Huff, 2007: 109).

Thus, the US regulatory environment allows businesses to have undue influence on the making and enforcement of the rules by which they are supposed to abide. Worse, even scientific "facts," the foundation of regulatory decisions, have become targets for industry influence seeking to deny links between a firm's product or production practices and health problems, in an effort to reduce the likelihood of litigation (Bohme et al., 2005: 338). A particularly audacious example involved industry ghost writing a paper published in the *Journal of Occupational and Environmental Medicine* when OSHA and the state of California were trying to set regulatory standards for chromium (VI). The article, was eventually exposed and retracted (Pearce, 2008).

As David Michaels (2008) has shown, seeding the scientific world with misleading information, pioneered by the tobacco industry's clouding of the scientific record on smoking and lung cancer, is now standard practice for US business. The techniques include funding studies that contradict the inconvenient scientific findings and hiring experts to cast doubt on the methods employed by the offending study. For example, in the 1960s when Irving Selikoff established the link between asbestos and cancer, the asbestos industry attempted to discredit it by claiming Selikoff's conclusions were "based on limited reports relating to a relatively small group of workers who install and/or remove a variety of insulation materials, including some which contain asbestos" (Bohme et al., 2005: 325). The industry also hired lawyers to write to Selikoff warning against "unwise" use of his research in public discussions, and claimed falsely after his death that Selikoff was a fraud because he had never obtained a medical degree (Bohme et al., 2005: 342). Taking advantage of the fundamental scientific principle of critical scrutiny, industry seeks to cast doubt where none should exist.

Public relations (PR) experts also play a role in industry's campaign against regulators. For example, in 1990 the PR firm ChemRisk worked for the American Petroleum Institute (API) to downplay the dangers of benzene, in part by developing "a succinct, yet scientifically compelling, integrated position statement to be used in comments to the state of North Carolina and as a possible springboard for future analyses that could be presented to US EPA and the State of California" (Bohme et al., 2005: 341). The list of products over which regulatory oversight was delayed or prevented altogether includes (but is by no means limited to) benzene, vinyl chloride, lead, asbestos, Vioxx, and arsenic (Michaels, 2008; see also Bohme et al., 2005; Huff, 2007; Pearce, 2008).

Industry can also set up and fund seemingly independent professional organizations, with suitably learned titles, as fronts for research that supports the corporate position, such as the Society for Toxicology, the Toxicology Forum, the American College of Toxicology, and the International Commission on Occupational Health (Huff, 2007: 109). Even the Chemical Industry Institute of Technology (CIIT), which clearly states that it "generates data which supports industry positions on risk analysis to modulate federal regulatory demands" (Bohme et al., 2005: 340), has been very successful in convincing the EPA that studies linking certain chemicals to cancer in animals are not applicable to humans (Bohme et al., 2005). It has argued that the burden of proof should come from epidemiological evidence, which would conveniently take 20 to 40 years to amass and can be contested even when it appears, as the tobacco industry did.

While industry makes powerful attempts to control its regulators, it need not always get its way, and regulation is a venue of conflict and debate. In a democratic society, citizens could vote for sweeping changes to the context in which firms operate. They could outlaw benzene, prevent junk food companies from advertising to children, and improve air quality. But all of these policies would impose costs on firms. As a result of the primacy of interests in the United States, the recent history of government involvement in public health has been less about protecting the public and more about promoting industry.

Citizens can also litigate to punish guilty firms and deter future harmful actions. However, the 1993 precedent-setting ruling in the case Daubert vs Merrell Dow Pharmaceuticals made this more difficult. A mother sued the drug firm because she blamed her child's birth defect on Bendectin, an anti-nausea drug. Her case was based on two pieces of evidence, animal tests that showed a link between the drug and birth anomalies, and human case studies where other users also had children with the same birth defect. In a sharp deviation from previous cases, the court ruled both types of evidence inadmissible for not being epidemiological studies that demonstrated harm in sufficient numbers of human subjects. Not only would establishing links that meet this burden of proof be difficult and take time, it can also be very challenging in a scientific world where the waters are increasingly muddied by corporate-funded influence. The result of this single, precedent-setting decision is that litigation has also become an increasingly unlikely venue for success in constraining corporate dangers.

Left to their own devices, firms will often take actions that harm people, whether they lead to unhealthy food, a polluted environment, or hazardous work. Since the 1980s the regulatory agencies that have been set up to shield people have become increasingly dominated by the corporations that they are supposed to be overseeing. As a result the chemicals in our food, environment, and workplaces are increasingly unmonitored, and their effects are unknown or downplayed. Although the regulatory decline has been a broad trend throughout the developed world, the extent of the decline is particular to the United States. Other nations in the world, with differing class relationships, have maintained a much stronger commitment to regulating the harmful health effects of modern capitalist enterprise. In fact, Chapter 6 will investigate the REACH regulation in Europe, which turned the regulatory burden of proof required in the United States on its head, requiring industry to demonstrate that products are safe rather than forcing the government to prove that they are harmful.

Labor market changes

As we have pointed out elsewhere, the US labor market has favored firms much more than their employees relative to other developed nations. Yet, the post Second World War period represented something of a high water mark for workers. The Wagner Act of 1935 guaranteed workers' right to organize and bargain collectively, leading to a wave of union formation especially during the war, when pressure to continue production and labor shortages created considerable power for workers. Low unemployment after the Second World War coupled with strong productivity increases and US global economic dominance created a unique situation in which US labor achieved considerable gains. It was during this period that US workers enjoyed steady wage increases that matched productivity gains (as we saw in Figure 3.1). It was also a period when inequality declined in the United States. However, this "golden age" of wage gains and declining inequality was not to last.

Public health was not only compromised by the decimation of regulatory protections that once at least partially sheltered people in the United States. The labor market has also become a much more uncertain, miserly, and undemocratic place, none of which is likely to improve health outcomes. Restructuring the labor market occurred over the same period, for the same reasons, and benefited the same group in society as the regulatory transformation. The decline in profitability for US firms was not only put down to the heavy hand of government regulation, it was also attributed to the high cost and sub-par performance of the slothful US worker. In an effort to reduce labor costs and increase profits, the United States embarked on a series of changes that would dramatically alter the power relationships between employer and employee.

The two major, and interrelated, tactics that firms employed to achieve these goals were moving the location of production, especially of labor-intensive manufactured goods, and changing labor market policy in the United States. Relocating production in search of lower costs was facilitated by free trade agreements, but was also possible within the United States, since individual states had drastically different labor market environments. Firms also successfully pressed for a change in domestic policies that would create what was euphemistically termed labor market flexibility, which in reality meant reducing the protections that US workers had fought for and won since the turn of the century. The labor market policies that were blamed for the supposed inferiority of the US workforce were the social supports like welfare funded by a progressive income tax, and rules favorable to unions. It was certainly true that these policies increased businesses' labor costs. In addition, a progressive tax structure in which the rich pay a larger percentage of their income tends to cost the well-to-do owners of capital more than those lower down the income ladder. The inevitable result of capital mobility in an environment of differing costs was that very real economic pressure was created for higher-cost areas to change their policies.

This is not a deterministic claim that wages and taxes will become equalized around the world as firms rush to produce only where labor costs are cheapest and environmental regulations the most lax. If this were the case, firms would be concentrating their production in the poorest countries, which is not happening for a number of reasons.

Many firms, in areas like resource extraction or services, are tied to a specific location. Other firms rely heavily on advanced technology and a skilled labor force, which can often only be found in more high-cost environments. Still other companies benefit from "clustering" around similar firms, as is the case in Silicon Valley (Porter, 2000). All of these factors mean that there can be different labor market policies in different areas without a lemming-like rush of firms out of the higher-cost area. Chapter 6 will show that a country like Sweden, with a much stronger labor movement, more extensive social welfare policies, and greater income equality than in the United States, is still one of the most competitive economies in the world. So, the damage done to the US workforce is not inevitable.

Labor force protections have been better maintained in other nations without a collapse in their competitive position. Yet this does not alter the underlying logic of the corporation, that where possible, lower costs are preferable. Sweden is not immune to downward pressure on its economic policies because its firms must also compete according to the profit-maximizing logic of capitalism. It has also restructured its economy, decreasing employment insurance benefits, for example, to increase labor market flexibility so it can stay competitive.

One example of the dramatic changes in the US labor market landscape during this period is the state of the union movement. Unions are much weaker in the United States than they are in many other developed nations. In part, this is because of laws, such as those outlawing solidarity strikes, which forced labor to "act as an interest group rather than a class" (Navarro, 1984: 521). Since the US working class cannot work as a collective whole, but as separate components, it has not achieved the broad protections or benefits enjoyed by its more unified Western European counterparts (Navarro, 1984: 521). Union membership has also fallen precipitously. Figure 4.6 shows the percentage of unionized workers in the United States. Although the union movement began to decline after its height of 34 percent in 1954, it declined more quickly after 1980 with the increased capital mobility and rule changes that made it more difficult to form and maintain unions. By 2010, membership stood at 11.9 percent of the working population. The withering of union membership in the United States has important public health implications beyond its obvious implications for wages and inequality. The demand–control model of workplace stress suggests that a lack of control over the workplace environment is one of the sources of poor health. A well-functioning union can provide

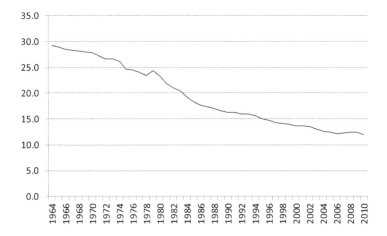

Figure 4.6 US unionization rate, percentage of nonagricultural wage and salary employees who are covered by collecting bargaining, 1964–2010

Source: Hirsch, Macpherson, and Vroman (2001: 51–5), plus accompanying data online at www.unionstats.com.

workers with an important venue to influence their employment conditions through a democratic process, and so gives them a greater "voice" in their work environment. The decline in union coverage can therefore be associated with a loss of a sense of control for many workers and an associated increase in stress.

As a result of all of these labor market changes, this period saw a shift in power from employees to employers, creating what former Federal Reserve Bank chairman Alan Greenspan has referred to as the "traumatized worker" in the United States.

> Increases in hourly compensation ... have continued to fall far short of what they would have been had historical relationships between compensation gains and the degree of labor market tightness held .... The continued reluctance of workers to leave their jobs to seek other employment as the labor market has tightened provides further evidence of such concern, as does the tendency toward longer labor union contracts. The low level of work stoppages of recent years also attests to concern about job security .... The continued decline in the state of the private workforce in labor unions has likely made wages more responsive to market forces .... Owing in part to the subdued behavior

of wages, profits and rates of return on capital has risen to high
levels.

(Greenspan, 1997)

It is these changes to the labor market that are responsible for the
inequality trends outlined earlier in the chapter. It is not only that
the rich are benefiting more from economic growth than the less well
off, but also that those who earn an income from capital are making
substantially more than those who earn income from labor. From 1973
to 1997, labor productivity grew by 29 percent in the United States, but
there was a decline in labor's share of corporate sector income and an
increase in profitability (Mishel, Bernstein, and Schmitt, 1999: 153–5).
According to Lester Thurow, US real per capita GDP rose 36 percent
from 1973 to 1995, yet the real hourly wages of nonsupervisory
workers declined by 14 percent. In the decade of the 1980s, all of the
earnings gains went to the top 20 percent of income earners, and an
amazing 64 percent to the already massively wealthy top 1 percent
(Thurow, 1996: 2). During this period, the average product per
worker grew significantly faster than wages, providing the profit and
motivation to invest. However, this also created growing inequality
and wage stagnation for the majority of the US working population.

For the privilege of a modest income, US workers were being
asked to work longer hours than their more fortunate developed
world contemporaries. In a dramatic turnaround, people in the
United States now work longer hours than the Japanese, who during
the 1980s were notorious for their commitment to their firms, and
whose intense work ethic was contrasted with US labor's less dutiful
approach to their work lives. According to Robert Reich, University
of California at Berkeley professor of public policy and former
secretary of labor under Bill Clinton, by the mid-2000s, US workers
were working an average of 2,200 hours per year, 350 more than the
average European (more than eight 40-hour weeks) (Reich, 2010:
62). Because there are only so many hours in the day, part of this
increased work time has come at the expense of sleep. People in the
United States now sleep between one and two hours less per night
than they did in the 1960s (Reich, 2010: 86).

The increase in individual hours understates the increase in paid
work time of US families since it does not account for the increase in
female labor force participation. In 1966 only 20 percent of women
with young children worked outside the home. That number rose
to 60 percent by the late 1990s. As a result, US families put in 500
more hours of paid work at the turn of the twenty-first century than

they did in 1979 (Reich, 2010: 62). The amount of hours that US workers put into their jobs is an indicator of the limited employment benefits that they get compared with other nations. Europeans get four or five weeks of leave by law and the Japanese have two legally mandated weeks, while the United States is the only industrialized nation with no minimum paid-leave law. Europeans have more generous provisions for sickness, compassionate leave, and parental time off. All of these measures decrease the insecurity and stress associated with balancing people's work and home lives.

The trends in the US labor market were moving in an ominous direction even before the economic collapse of 2008, which caused the unemployment rate to balloon from 4 to 10 percent. The restructuring of the labor market had the effect of transferring power from workers to employers. As a result, jobs have become less secure, less democratic, and there are longer hours and fewer benefits. In a not unrelated development, the income of most workers in the United States has increased only marginally, if at all, during this period while the income shares at the very top have gone up dramatically. The evidence presented earlier in this chapter proved that there are strong relationships between a wide variety of negative health results and jobs that are insecure, lack control, and are not sufficiently rewarding. Evidence also connects growing inequality to a host of problematic health results. Yet, this is precisely the path taken by the United States since 1980. As was the case with regulation, the United States is an exception in terms of its labor market policy, resulting from its uniquely weak working class and the particularly strong influence of business. While subject to the same economic pressures as the United States, other nations have more successfully maintained labor market policies that create a better balance between the interests of workers and their employers. Chapter 6 will examine the more egalitarian labor market policies of Sweden as one example.

CONCLUSION

The US economy has historically been remarkably innovative. Dramatic productivity increases (and the ability of the laboring population to glean a stable portion of that increase) permitted the country to escape the burden of infectious disease and early death. Yet those productivity gains contained their own costs in terms of public health, creating health problems for the food we eat, the air we breathe, and the conditions in which we work and the products we consume. This is not to suggest that our times are not an improvement on the grim days of old. However, there is a sizeable gap between what exists and what would be possible if we paid much closer attention to how the profit motive has shaped the conditions in which we live. The increasing corporate colonization of science and the regulatory agencies that once provided at least a modicum of protection has made the situation graver still.

A similar point can be made in relation to work. There are fewer grim industrial accidents, wages have increased, and social protection is greater than in the early industrial United States. Yet, work still contains unnecessary dangers to human health. The dangers are more pronounced for those in the lower echelons, in terms of both income and work hierarchy. The United States is the most unequal developed nation in the world, and has one of the most insecure and stressed labor forces. While between 1950 and 1970 things were much better on this front, starting in 1980 the sweeping changes to the labor market that changed the power relationships between workers and owners resulted in a redistribution of income to the top of the income spectrum and created a more insecure, impoverished existence for a generation of US workers.

The best explanation for chronic disease is to be found in the interaction of distress, fat, cholesterol, tobacco, chemicals, and economic inequality, all of which are the products of historically specific socially determined production and distribution conditions, created by twentieth-century capitalism. We are most certainly not alone in this claim. In 2009, Jason Beckfield and Nancy Krieger appealed for increased attention to the social factors in health, arguing that:

> neither the forms of social inequality nor their associations with health status are "fixed" but instead are historically contingent. Moreover, recognizing the interplay between the embodied facts of health inequities and how they are conceptualized, ecosocial theory also calls attention to accountability and agency, both for social inequalities in health and for ways they are—or are not— monitored, analyzed, and addressed.
>
> (Beckfield and Krieger, 2009: 153)

This call was mirrored by a 2008 report by the World Health Organization (WHO) Commission on the Social Determinants of Health, which argues that health is shaped by the conditions in which "people grow, work, live and age." As the WHO points out in its executive summary, "social justice is a matter of life and death" (2008b: 1).

5

THE POLITICAL ECONOMY OF US HEALTHCARE: THE MEDICAL INDUSTRIAL COMPLEX

> Of all the forms of inequality, injustice in health care is the most shocking and inhumane.
>
> (Martin Luther King Jr. in a speech to the Medical Committee for Human Rights, 1966)

In 2012, the local Minnesota press picked up what, on the surface, was a feel-good story. Stacy Knudson, a 43-year-old waitress working the midnight shift at the Fryn' Pan, received a $12,000 tip in a shoebox full of rolled-up cash. After the suspicious local constabulary determined that the money was not needed as evidence in a drug trial and let Knudson keep the cash, she claimed that it was "a complete miracle to see our prayers answered." Knudson was not going to use the money for a new car or a lavish vacation, but to pay off the family's medical bills. In the past year her husband had been hurt at work and she had fractured her knee. Before the cash windfall, she had being trying to pay the bills by working two part-time jobs in addition to her late-night gig at the local diner (Oakes and Norfleet, 2012). To observers in every other wealthy country, this story would be patently absurd and slightly tragic. What sort of healthcare system would force people to rely on divine intervention to meet their medical expenses?

The broad social and environmental conditions in which people live and work may be the primary determinants of people's health, but it is the healthcare system that deals with the consequences of those conditions. A well-functioning healthcare system can play a vital role in improving the quality of life for people. While choosing the right car might be a source of pride or frustration, getting the right diagnosis and medical intervention, or even being able to see someone capable of providing a diagnosis, can be a matter of comfort or pain, and in extreme cases life or death. When people are not able to access reliable care it is rightly taken to be an important failing not only of the healthcare system but of a society's ability to care for its citizens.

The type of healthcare system in a country will have a large impact on people's access to care, and the quality of care within the system. When people think of the healthcare system, they usually think about their doctor. Yet the healthcare system comprises a much larger web of goods and services, including many that are behind the scenes from the user's perspective, including insurance, drugs, hospitals, clinics, and laboratories. All of these can be owned in a variety of ways including state, private non-profits, private independent, and corporate. The healthcare system in most countries is a mixture of different types of ownership. In the United Kingdom, the National Health Service established in 1948 was a single-payer, universal healthcare system, where hospitals were owned by the state. In Canada, hospitals are independent non-profits, where most medical services are paid for and financed by the state through universal public insurance. In the United States, hospitals are run by for-profit corporations, non-profits, and even the state through the Veterans Administration. Health insurance is provided through the pubic Medicare and Medicaid programs, employer-based insurance, and private schemes. Many people also pay directly for their own care.

There are two key differences between the United States and the rest of the industrialized world. First, the United States is alone in the developed world in eschewing a government-led or regulated plan of universal insurance coverage. In every other industrialized country there is a guarantee that, no matter how the rest of the healthcare system is owned and organized, its citizens will have complete coverage for necessary physician and hospital services. All of these other nations have deliberately removed access to healthcare from the realm of the market. The logic behind this, at its most fundamental level, is that access to medical services should not be determined by an individual's ability to pay either directly for the health services or through insurance premiums. The second difference is that the United States relies more heavily on the private, for-profit sector to deliver its healthcare. This chapter attempts to explain why the United States has evolved a more market-driven, for-profit system than the rest of the developed world, and to outline some of the problematic consequences of this "exceptionalism."

The United States has not developed its unique structure because it was the "popular choice," although some have made this claim. Perhaps most famously detailed in Paul Starr's 1982 book *The Social Transformation of American Medicine*, the argument is that the US healthcare system evolved in its particular form, including the lack of universal public health insurance, because that is what people want (see also Ginzberg, 1977: 3; Fein, 1986; Fuchs, 1986: 269). So the healthcare system is a legitimate expression of the beliefs and values of the majority of US citizens as both consumers and voters. This confident assertion rests on a couple of crucial and questionable assumptions. First, it begs the question of just how the beliefs and values of people are formed. It is possible that the formation of beliefs is a result of the current system rather than the other way around. The commonly held beliefs in any society are not a result of people selecting what they consider to be the best option out of a menu of ideas that compete on a level playing field. Rather, the formation of beliefs, and the ideas that influence them, are a product of powerful interests that are better able to get their ideas disseminated to the public. Second, it assumes that popular wishes get translated into public policy. Yet polling data shows that the US population repeatedly and consistently favored a universal, comprehensive health program, even if it resulted in higher taxes, but this has not been translated into political action (Navarro, 1989).

It is clear that people in the United States are not getting the healthcare system they want. As we have done in previous chapters, we will suggest that the US healthcare system is a product of a political and economic conflict between differing classes in society with very different, and often conflicting, interests. The first section provides a brief history of how these different interests have shaped the evolution of healthcare in the United States. The second section analyses the US healthcare system in terms of access and efficiency. The third section exposes the flaws in the intellectual justifications for the private, for-profit system in the United States. Finally, Obama's healthcare reform package is explained in light of our class-based theory of US healthcare policy.

CLASS INTERESTS: THE EVOLUTION OF THE MEDICAL INDUSTRIAL COMPLEX

A private health-care industry of huge proportions could be a powerful political force in the country and could exert considerable influence on national health policy. A broad national health-insurance program, with the inevitable federal regulation of costs, would be anathema to the medical-industrial complex, just as a national disarmament policy is to the military-industrial complex.

(Relman, 1980: 969)

Like the conditions of work and the state of the environment, the healthcare system is influenced by the outcome of the conflict between groups with opposing interests. US healthcare has been shaped by the conflict between the general public's dissatisfaction with the private system and those who have a vested interest in that system. As we shall see in the following section, the specific mechanisms through which this conflict played out, and the specific groups that took the lead for each side, changed over time. However, this did not change the constant that a weak working class failed to win universal public health insurance in the face of a well-organized, powerful medical industry. In this conflict between US citizens and a specific faction of US industry, the broader business class, which once sided with the medical industry, has become more ambivalent in its support in recent years because of changing economic circumstances. The domination of US healthcare by the medical industry has resulted in an unresolved contradiction. What is desired by the industry has not been satisfactory to the general public. This has manifested itself in serious demands for universal health insurance five times in the 1900s.

The early years: the AMA

In the early decades of the 1900s, the forces of progressive reform called for expanded access to healthcare. In Europe, workers, their union organizations and the political parties that represented them were the driving force behind universal public insurance (see Table 5.1). Between 1883 and 1910 every Western European nation passed some form of sickness insurance (Hacker, 2002: 193). In these nations, the labor movement pressed for universal, healthcare systems with very specific characteristics. First, they wanted a universal, as opposed to means tested, or targeted, system. Second, they insisted on labor movement input into the direction of the healthcare system. Third, the state was to be in financial control of the system. Finally, it should be funded through a system of progressive income tax (Navarro, 1989). This structure contained two important principles for European workers: solidarity and redistribution. By making a uniform level of benefits

Table 5.1 Establishment of major trade union federations, socialist parties and first social (including health) insurance: selected European countries

Country	Trade union	Socialist party	Social insurance
United Kingdom	1868	1900	1908
Germany	1868	1875	1883
Sweden	1898	1889	1913

Source: (Navarro 1989: 140).

available to the entire population, the unity of the labor movement was strengthened. Simultaneously, it strengthened the populations' commitment to public healthcare since the benefits did not only go to an unfortunate (or undeserving) minority of poor families, but to the entire population. Funding through progressive income tax was a deliberate strategy to redistribute income from high-earning business owners to lower-earning workers. Why were European workers able to get their demands for public health insurance implemented while US workers repeatedly failed in the United States?

It was not as though there was no pressure for health insurance in the United States. In 1912, Theodore Roosevelt endorsed compulsory health insurance. In 1916, the American Association for Labor Legislation pushed for health insurance at the state level. Both of these proposals failed, while similar proposals in Europe succeeded. Vicente Navarro (1989) makes a convincing case that one of the major reasons for this difference is that, despite the increased strength of the working class in the United States during the Progressive period, it was still relatively much weaker than European labor. The percentage of unionized workers in the United States is lower than in Europe. For much of US history, unions were organized along weaker, more conservative craft lines, as opposed to industrial unions, and had no centralized bargaining process. US labor has never had a significant political party to represent working-class interests. As a result, any popular demands for a universal public system could not be channeled through established union organizations or political parties. In fact, the AFL, the largest union organization in the late 1800s and early 1900s, openly opposed any kind of publically funded healthcare. The notoriously conservative president of the AFL, Samuel Gompers, was concerned that public healthcare (and any other government protection for that matter, from minimum wage to unemployment insurance) would diminish the influence of unions, since one of the principal benefits that unions could offer their members would be removed from the negotiating table and placed in the hands of the state (Starr, 1982: 250).

While the US population did not have a ready vehicle to push forward its demands for health insurance, the opposition was unified and well organized. In contrast to workers' compensation, where employers were divided because many could see a potential benefit through a reduction in legal settlements arising from injuries at work, business could see no similar gains from public health insurance. Business groups were opposed to a public system because they were against public intervention in principle, concerned about being forced to pay for a public program, predicted it would create an increase in employee "malingering," and because they were worried that it would decrease employee loyalty to the firm that was created by employer-funded insurance (Hoffman, 2001: 113–14). From the workers' perspective, this "employee loyalty" was generated by the additional insecurity that came with losing health coverage along with their job. Universal public insurance that would guarantee coverage even to those without work would reduce employers' power in the labor market. The medical industry provided the vanguard of the opposition to compulsory health insurance. Although health insurance was in its infancy at this time, the insurance companies of Prudential and Metropolitan lobbied to prevent a national insurance program, worried that it would cut into their lucrative trade in life insurance which offered the working class a way of avoiding the dreaded "pauper's burial." During this period the drug companies also lined up in opposition out of concern that a government-run program would have considerable bargaining power over the price of pharmaceutical products.

The most vocal opposition to health insurance came from the American Medical Association (AMA). Although it originally provided tentative support for the social reformers who wanted a national universal health insurance program in the 1910s, support was withdrawn over concerns that it eliminated doctors' discretion over their fees, and that fees for services would be changed to a salary or capitation system (a fixed sum per patient per year) under national insurance. One Buffalo doctor claimed that health insurance would create a "heartless, overworked, 15 cent-a-call contract physician" (Hoffman, 2001: 89). After its early flirtation with universal healthcare, the AMA led the opposition to any intrusion into its professional domain.

As we saw in Chapter 2, the early decades of the twentieth century witnessed the formalization of the medical profession, part of which was the growing strength of its association. By 1930, 65 percent of doctors belonged to the AMA. By 1920, it issued a declaration opposed to any "system of compulsory contribution insurance" that was "provided, controlled or regulated" by the government (Hacker, 2002: 198). Indeed, at this point, doctors were also opposed to private, voluntary insurance, which they feared would interfere with their professional purview. Similar class alignments thwarted the next wave of health insurance proposals in the 1930s and 1940s. In 1935, health insurance was proposed as part of the New Deal that ushered in Social Security but was left out of the final Act. In the late 1940s the Wagner–Murray–Dingwall Bill, which would have introduced public universal insurance, also failed.

The two major changes of this period were the growing strength of US workers and the fledgling development of the private health insurance industry. The pressure for reform again came from popular demands to ensure access to healthcare as the costs of medical care began to increase, in part because of the formalization and direction imposed by the Flexner Report (see Chapter 2). In 1943, 85 percent of people in the United States favored a system of healthcare modeled on Social Security. As organized labor moved to a more inclusive form of industrial unionism, it supported universal public health. However, this support was not unequivocal. Although the Congress of Industrial Organizations (CIO) decried voluntary insurance in 1949, and provided surface support for public insurance in the 1930s and 1940s, it made little concrete effort to win public, universal health insurance through political means. This was especially true after the Taft Hartley Act of 1947 purged unions of their more radical leaders, tactics, and ambitions. Public insurance would strip one of the fringe benefits that bread and butter unionism could use to attract workers in the more hostile post-Taft Hartley environment (Quadagno, 2004: 31). While the union movement was the driving force behind universal public insurance in other nations, in the United States its efforts were channeled into getting private insurance through collective bargaining.

Without the driving force of a fully committed union movement, public desire for universal public health insurance could not overcome entrenched opposition spearheaded by the AMA, which followed a two-pronged approach. The first was to decry any public insurance. The AMA levied a $25 fee on its members for an unprecedented multi-million-dollar campaign in the late 1940s, billing public insurance as a communist plot to bring "socialism" to the United States which would result in "low-grade assembly line medicine" (Quadagno, 2004: 30). It communicated its position through letter-writing campaigns, newspaper ads, and personal letters from doctors to their patients. In addition to shaping public opinion, it directly campaigned against politicians who were proposing public plans (Hacker, 2002: 225; Quadagno, 2004: 30). The AMA drew support from the other medical industry groups like the American Hospital Association (AHA), insurance companies, and drug manufacturers. Organizations representing the broader business class, like the Chamber of Commerce, also publically opposed any government intrusion into private healthcare profits.

The second prong was to offer private insurance as a deliberate tactic to ease the political pressure for the more odious, as far as the AMA was concerned, public alternative. In 1940 only 6 million people in the United States had any kind of medical insurance, but the figure expanded over 12 times, to 75 million by the end of the decade (Quadagno, 2004). Private insurance was palatable to doctors, in part because the medical profession was in control of early insurance organizations. First, the AHA (Blue Cross) and then the AMA (Blue Shield) set up non-profit organizations that offered early forms of voluntary insurance, but in a manner that avoided the medical profession's concern about third-party intervention in its professional decisions (Quadagno, 2004: 30). In some ways, hospitals even benefited from insurance. Early Blue Cross policies were, in effect, a prepayment for hospital services, where families would pay a monthly fee in exchange for free hospital stays of a certain length. For hospitals, this increased the number of patients that could use their services and created a smooth, predictable revenue flow. While business was not keen on the increasing costs of employer-based health insurance, it preferred the voluntary private form of insurance over the public option. Like the paternalistic corporate efforts implemented in the Progressive period, firms felt that it would increase employee loyalty. This was especially true during the Second World War when wage controls encouraged firms to offer fringe benefits to attract employees in a tight labor market (Quadagno, 2004: 31).

The failure of public insurance did not mean that government was not involved in healthcare spending. Rather, it was heavily involved, but in a manner that was amenable to the profitability of the private healthcare sector. In 1946, the Hospital Survey and Construction Act (or Hill–Burton Act) provided grants and loans for healthcare facility construction and modernization (Hoffman,

2001: 183). In exchange for this financial help, facilities had to offer a "reasonable volume" of services to area residents who would not otherwise be able to pay for medical care. The enforcement of the reasonable volume provisions was virtually nonexistent in the early years of this Act, meaning that those who could not pay did not necessarily get access to Hill–Burton funded hospitals. Yet the bill did permit the medical establishment to claim that it was increasing access for poorer members of the community, while increasing the supply of medical facilities in the country.

After the defeat of Wagner–Murray–Dingwall, the employer-based system was firmly entrenched as the dominant method of insurance. Doctors, hospitals, insurance companies, and employers all benefited from private insurance. On top of this it had the added political bonus of neutralizing the demand for public insurance. Unions may have paid lip service to a public option, but their energies were dedicated to expanding private insurance to their members. The supremacy of private insurance was further supported by the 1954 tax code change that made employer contributions to worker health plans tax exempt, a policy supported by the AMA and AHA. It was also supported by the CIO despite the fact that it would clearly benefit rich workers more than poor, and only those workers with employer coverage (Hacker, 2002: 204). As a result of these changes, the percentage of people covered by private insurance in the United States grew from 10 percent in 1940 to 70 percent in 1960 (Hacker, 2002: 214).

The passage of Medicare Part A in 1965, which ensures hospital care, demonstrated both the promise of collective, popular action and its limits. Medicare was passed because of pressure from the elderly and the AFL-CIO, despite a strong counter campaign by the AMA, showing that the entrenched interests of the medical industry were not all-powerful. Yet it is worth noting that insurance companies were not strongly opposed to Medicare because they felt that the elderly "would never be profitable" (Quadagno, 2004: 32). Rather than opposing Medicare, insurance companies successfully lobbied to carve out a profitable niche in the program, which they achieved when Medicare left many health needs uncovered and passage of Part B of the bill allowed private companies to insure physician services. The AMA and AHA managed to get guarantees that the government would not use its public insurance to control doctor or hospital fees. Further, the impact of achieving public insurance for the largest remaining identifiable group of uninsured in the United States reduced the demand for true universal coverage. It is worth noting that it was during the late 1960s, while the United States limited itself to public insurance for the elderly, its economically similar northern neighbors in Canada achieved universal public coverage through the demands of a new social democratic party.

Modern America: insurance and corporate medicine

Medicare and Medicaid (partial state coverage for the poor) may have papered over the worst of the cracks in the private, employer-based system, but rising medical costs and public dissatisfaction soon caused them to reappear. Business was concerned about the growing cost of insurance. Labor was dissatisfied with increasing insurance premiums and declining employee benefits, as firms attempted to pass insurance costs on to their workers. The government also grew increasingly disenchanted with the growing expense of funding the hybrid health insurance system. The cost of the private health insurance tax exemption alone rose to $110 billion by the late 1990s and about $130 billion in 2006. The increasing resentment about the employer-based system of insurance came as the AMA was replaced by the rapidly growing private insurance industry as the protector of private medicine. Any demands for universal insurance would have to either overcome or accommodate the demands of the increasingly powerful insurance industry and its colleagues in an increasingly corporate medical delivery system.

It was in this context that Clinton's Health Security (HS) plan was introduced in 1993. The plan was not for public insurance. Rather, it would provide universal access through employer-mandated private insurance offering managed care, which gives insurance companies control over healthcare providers. Despite this concession, the insurance industry opposed the final bill because of proposed increased regulation and cost control (Navarro, 2007). It was the insurance industry, rather than the AMA, that now took the lead in defeating HS. The Health Insurance Association of America (HIAA) spent lavishly on advertising to sway public opinion, political donations, and lobbying. The HIAA also drew support from small businesses, which stood to lose more than their larger contemporaries since many of them did not offer insurance to their employees (Hacker, 2002: 264; Quadagno, 2004: 38).

Dissatisfaction with HS was easy to generate. Neither the labor movement nor social movements like Public Citizen, which collected 200,000 signatures in support of a single payer system (Navarro, 2007), were particularly enamored of the managed care option. In fact, the insurance-directed managed care alternative in the HS would have likely amounted to "assembly line" healthcare for the masses (Navarro, 2007). Given that the existing system had created its own constituents through Medicare and employer-based insurance, people had legitimate questions about whether HS would actually improve their access to health. The Clinton plan was doomed to failure. Its futile attempt to accommodate the insurance industry resulted in an at best mediocre insurance plan for the public, which failed to generate any constituency that would support it while still managing to create opposition from the insurance industry and business groups that it tried so hard to placate.

The defeat of Clinton's plan meant that the problems of US healthcare continued to escalate. The majority of the population continued to resent the existing system. In 2007, seven separate polls showed that the majority of people in the United States were in favor of a universal government plan. For example, a 2007 Associated Press poll found that 54 percent of respondents answered "yes," while 44 percent answered "no" to this question: "Do you consider yourself a supporter of a single-payer healthcare system, that is a national health plan financed by taxpayers in which all Americans would get their insurance from a single government plan, or not?" Similar results were found in polls conducted by the National Small Business Association (60 percent in favor), and CBS (55 percent in favor) to name a couple of the other examples. In the run-up to Obama's healthcare plan a *New York Times* poll found that 72 percent of the population preferred a public plan (Hilzenrath, 2009).

Despite business attempts to get out from under health costs, employer insurance remained the backbone of the insurance system for the non-elderly. About 63 percent of the under-65 population were still covered through their work in 2006. The amount that large firms were paying for healthcare was genuinely staggering. Prior to the economic crisis, and the auto industry restructuring in 2008, General Motors spent $5 billion on healthcare each year, or about $1,500–$2,000 per car, far more than in other nations (Johnson, 2010). It is not only the automobile industry that is concerned with health costs. By 2005, Starbucks was spending $200 million a year in health insurance, more than it was spending on coffee beans. Wal-Mart has only insured around half of its employees, but it still spent $1.5 billion on health insurance for its US workers (Picard, 2005).

As a result, there are signs that business is organizing to lobby for changes that would reduce its healthcare costs. The Washington Business Group on Health has evolved to lobby for some form of cost control in corporate healthcare expenses (Starr, 1982: 444). Business groups now support regulation of health insurance premiums. Business leaders have even joined the National Coalition on Health Care (NCHC), which supports universal coverage, cost management, improved healthcare quality, equitable financing, and simplified administration (Geyman, 2003: 322). This is not the same as supporting a publicly funded, single-payer scheme. In fact the NCHC's goal is to create "a truly competitive health care marketplace" (NCHC, 2009). What it does reveal is the inherent conflict facing businesses on this issue.

While the interests of the business community as a whole might be ambiguous on this issue, there is one corporate sector that is unequivocally and vociferously opposed to reducing the for-profit component of the healthcare system. The term medical industrial complex (MIC) was first used in Barbara and John Ehrenreich's (1971) *The American Health Empire* to highlight the fact that the primary purpose of healthcare corporations is not to improve people's health, but to make profits. It described the profitable link between doctors, hospitals, and medical schools on one hand, and the more corporate side of the industry such as insurance companies, drug manufacturers, and medical equipment suppliers on the other. As early as the 1980s, industry observers were warning about a "new" MIC to signify the increasing corporate control of sectors of the industry that were either non-profit, state-owned, or small-scale for-profit like hospitals and labs (Relman, 1980). In the evolved MIC, larger conglomerates have non-profit and for-profit components, "rendering impossible the simple differentiation of public from private" (Estes, Harrington, and Pellow, 2000: 1,825). Yet there is little question that growth is a fundamental dynamic of the for-profit corporate sector, which will, in the absence of outside constraints, lead to its expansion over time. In *Medicine and Public Health at the End of Empire*, Howard Waitzkin (2011) demonstrates that the profit-maximizing requirements of multinational medical firms can explain much of the evolution of healthcare systems around the world, including the dramatic expansion of coronary care units in the United States despite a worrying lack of clinical evidence for their effectiveness (Waitzkin, 2011: 28–30). So the MIC is a combination of the old and the new, with the well-established players in industries like drugs and insurance joined by relative newcomers such as for-profit hospitals, lab services, and nursing home corporations. It is important to recognize that even a not-for-profit hospital can be an important conduit for generating profits for the MIC because it uses its drugs and technology. The division is further blurred because often the boards of non-profit hospitals overlap with the boards of for-profit companies that supply them.

The MIC has been fairly consistent in its opposition to public intrusion into the healthcare system in any form other than subsidization. The health insurance industry has been predictably hostile to what would be, at a minimum, a significant encroachment into its very profitable business. As the healthcare system becomes more corporatized, it is likely to increasingly resist proposals for nationalization of profitable sectors. For example, profit-making hospitals currently benefit from private health insurance, and

---

Humana

The rise of Humana is a nice example of how the medical industry has changed over the last 40 years. In 1968, Humana started its operations with a small handful of nursing homes in Louisville, Kentucky that earned $4.8 million. By 1980, it owned 92 hospitals and made $1.4 billion in revenues (Starr, 1982: 431). By 2010 it had expanded again, into the insurance business, with over 10 million people enrolled in its benefit plans. It employed 1,800 sales representatives and a further 800 telemarketers to advertise its insurance products, and owned over 300 medical centers, some of which are stationed in Wal-Mart thanks to a strategic partnership. Humana employed 1,900 medical professionals at its Concentra medical centers. Annual revenues for 2010 were $34 billion (Humana, 2011).

However, Humana's rise also highlights why some people question the benefits of for-profit institutions in healthcare. A 1980 *Fortune* article claimed that Humana would happily accept Medicaid and Medicare patients when it had empty beds to fill, but when it was running at closer to capacity it gave preferential treatment to the privately insured because it could bill them at a higher rate. The corporation also looks for the most profitable locations in which to locate its medical centers. Unsurprisingly, this is not in poorer areas, with a lower percentage of fully insured patients, but in suburbs with young, healthy, employed families. Indeed, the brutally cold logic of the company's for-profit orientation could not have been more clearly revealed than when an uninsured patient was transferred after suffering a heart attack and later died, and a Humana official commented, "These freebies cost $2000 to $3000 a day. Who's going to pay for them?" (Starr, 1982: 436).

would obviously oppose any reduction in the number of for-profit hospitals (Starr, 1982: 448). There is not inevitably an antagonism between the interests of all the components of the MIC and public health insurance, which can actually encourage for-profit sectors of the health industry by guaranteeing revenues. For example, when Medicare for the elderly was introduced in 1965 it resulted in a tremendous expansion in for-profit nursing homes (Starr, 1982: 445).

Many doctors have also supported national health programs. Recently, 64 percent of the American Medical Women's Association supported a single-payer plan, and Physicians for a National Health Program, which advocates a single-payer, national health insurance, boasts a membership of 18,000 (Geyman, 2003: 323). Yet, the AMA (with 250,000 members) is not in favor of a single-payer public plan, preferring instead to recommend that people "purchase the health insurance of their choice," with some financial assistance for low-income families. In a submission to the Senate Finance Committee, it wrote, "The introduction of a new public plan threatens to restrict patient choice by driving out private insurers, which currently provide coverage for nearly 70 percent of Americans" (Pear, 2009). Although the MIC is not a completely homogeneous group with respect to its interests in state intervention, it is a fairly accurate generalization that the MIC is in favor of government subsidies that increase the profits of private firms but opposes any state role in owning, regulating or negotiating prices in the industry.

The MIC's opposition takes many forms in order to sway both the public, in general, and politicians more specifically, to maintain the current private, for-profit system. The most direct way in which this occurs is through lobbying and donating to politicians. The MIC has spent lavishly in this area. In the 2008 presidential election, the finance, insurance, and real estate (FIRE) sector was the largest industry group donor, contributing $133 million, $71 million of which went to the Democrats. The health industry contributed an additional $42 million (Center for Responsive Politics, 2009). In the 2009–10 elections, the insurance industry contributed $42 million, health professionals an impressive $75 million and pharmaceuticals/health products an additional $31 million (Centre for Responsive Politics, 2010). Three of the top eleven sectors donating in the 2009–10 election were part of the MIC.

The MIC is consistently among the most active spenders in the US political system. Of course, not all of this money is dedicated to opposing public insurance. The MIC has to defend its interests over a wide range of public policies from drug testing and patent length in the pharmaceutical industry to protecting doctors from litigation. Yet in these examples as well, we can see the conflict that exists between the interests of the MIC and the general public. Only the most naïve of observers would expect this kind of money not to influence the policy decisions of politicians. Indeed, if it did not create influence, the profit-maximizing firms in the MIC would be throwing money away, which is an unacceptable conclusion.

The political influence of the MIC is also enhanced because there is a revolving door between high-level government positions and industry insiders. Often former government officials can count on jobs as healthcare industry lobbyists. Billy Tauzin spent 25 years in the House of Representatives. Among his accomplishments was to champion the 2003 Medicare Modernization Act which guaranteed large overpayments for private insurers and prevented Medicare from using its bargaining power to lower drug prices. Coincidentally, he left political office to become the president of PhRMA, a drug company lobbying firm (Krugman, 2009).

In 2009, 350 former members of Congress and government staff were under contract to lobby for insurance, hospital, or medical groups. Just to provide one example, Richard Tarplin worked for both the Department of Health and Human Services and Democratic Senator Christopher Dodd before opening his own lobbying firm, which represents the AMA. He describes how his experience in government can benefit his clients: "For people like me who are on the outside and used to be on the inside, this is great, because there is a level of trust in these relationships, and I know the policy rationale that is required" (Eggan and Kindy, 2009). Of course, the movement is both ways. A board member of a for-profit dialysis company that earns the bulk of its money from Medicare and Medicaid, Da Vita, became the chair of the Health Care Financing Administration (HCFA) that administers Medicare and Medicaid. At the same time, two HCFA administrators moved to senior positions at Da Vita (Geyman, 2003: 319). Seeding high levels of government health agencies with industry representatives will predictably result in the perspectives of the MIC being shared by those in government.

In a democracy, the opinions of the public can actually matter. As a result, the MIC has dedicated considerable time and effort to swaying people's opinions on the healthcare issue. It does so in a wide variety of ways from direct advertising to funding think tanks and academic positions. A particularly revealing exposé of the tactics employed by the MIC can be found in Wendell Potter's book *Deadly Spin*. As the former chief of public relations for health insurance company Cigna, Potter has an insider's view of the industry's efforts to influence the debate around public insurance. When Clinton was proposing healthcare reform in 1994 the insurance industry funded a $14 million advertising campaign in which "Harry and Louise," two burdened everyday suburbanites, lamented the state of a hypothetical future government health program run by bureaucrats with the tagline "when they choose we lose" (Singer, 2009: B3).

When documentary filmmaker Michael Moore released his 2007 critique of the state of US healthcare, *Sicko*, the health insurance (mis-)information service again sprang into action. Because Moore's film compared the US healthcare system unfavorably with the public insurance systems of Canada and Europe, the industry was concerned that it might sow disenchantment with private insurance. In response, it hired one of Washington's biggest PR firms to portray "Moore as someone intent on destroying the free-market health care system and with it, the American way of life" (Potter, 2010: 39). One tactic in the campaign was to set up and finance a fake grassroots campaign (or Astroturf in PR speak) called Health Care America to attack *Sicko* and the broader idea of a national, single-payer insurance plan (Potter, 2010: 37). These are not isolated examples. One healthcare expert summarized the state of debate on healthcare reform in the following manner: "There have been five well-motivated and serious attempts to enact a system of universal coverage in the United States over the last 100 years. On each occasion, health care stakeholders have pulled no punches in using disinformation and obfuscation to confuse and mislead the public" (Geyman, 2003: 316).

The unique healthcare system in the United States is not a result of the will of the people, in any meaningful sense. Rather, it is the result of a political battle between a relatively weak and disorganized working class, without any meaningful political representation, against a very well-funded and organized section of the corporate world, with an enormous stake in the continuation and expansion of a profit-making healthcare industry: the MIC. "What has become clear is that the unique problems the U.S. medical-industrial complex has created are rooted in the subordination of the state and civil society to corporate interests" (Estes et al., 2000: 1,827). It was in this less than favorable context that President Obama launched his effort at healthcare reform. As we shall see later in this chapter, the results were predictably disappointing.

Selections from the Testimony of Wendell Potter, Philadelphia, PA, before the US Senate Committee on Commerce, Science and Transportation, June 24, 2009

My name is Wendell Potter and for 20 years, I worked as a senior executive at health insurance companies, and I saw how they confuse their customers and dump the sick—all so they can satisfy their Wall Street investors.

I know from personal experience that members of Congress and the public have good reason to question the honesty and trustworthiness of the insurance industry. Insurers make promises they have no intention of keeping, they flout regulations designed to protect consumers, and they make it nearly impossible to understand—or even to obtain—information we need. As you hold hearings and discuss legislative proposals over the coming weeks, I encourage you to look very closely at the role for-profit insurance companies play in making our healthcare system both the most expensive and one of the most dysfunctional in the world. I hope you get a real sense of what life would be like for most of us if the kind of so-called reform the insurers are lobbying for is enacted.

To help meet Wall Street's relentless profit expectations, insurers routinely dump policyholders who are less profitable or who get sick....Why? Because dumping a small number of enrollees can have a big effect on the bottom line. Ten percent of the population accounts for two-thirds of all healthcare spending. The Energy and Commerce Committee's investigation into three insurers found that they cancelled the coverage of roughly 20,000 people in a five-year period, allowing the companies to avoid paying $300 million in claims.

They also dump small businesses whose employees' medical claims exceed what insurance underwriters expected. All it takes is one illness or accident among employees at a small business to prompt an insurance company to hike the next year's premiums so high that the employer has to cut benefits, shop for another carrier, or stop offering coverage altogether—leaving workers uninsured. The practice is known in the industry as purging....

The industry and its backers are using fear tactics, as they did in 1994, to tar a transparent, publicly accountable healthcare option as a government-run system. But what we have today, Mr. Chairman, is a Wall Street-run system that has proven itself an untrustworthy partner to its customers, to the doctors and hospitals who deliver care, and to the state and federal governments that attempt to regulate it.

THE RESULTS OF THE DOMINANCE OF THE MIC

The insurance industry

The health of US citizens has been poorer, the number of underinsured and uninsured individuals higher, and the cost of care greater than in any other industrialized nation. The US healthcare system's greater emphasis on private insurance and service delivery means that it fares poorly compared with other similar nations in terms of both access and efficiency.

Access to healthcare is largely determined by insurance coverage. While it is possible for patients to pay for care out of pocket, the expense of many procedures means that insurance is the only genuinely viable alternative for most people. The most commonly cited criticism of the US system prior to the Obama reform was that it denied healthcare to many of its citizens who lacked insurance. It was not the poorest who lacked coverage, since they were at least partially insured through the government-funded Medicaid program; rather, it was the people who were not quite poor enough to qualify for Medicaid yet did not have a job through which they could access health insurance. While it might be thought that this only described a few people who fell through the cracks in the system, in fact it was not an insignificant number. In 2007, prior to the Obama reforms, about 15–16 percent of the US population (over 40 million people) did not have insurance (DeNavas-Walt, Proctor, and Smith, 2008: 19). This only counts people who are uninsured for the entire year. Counting people who were without insurance for part of the year would add another 82 million to this number (Families USA, 2004). The number of people covered by employer-based programs was also falling as firms attempted to reduce their rapidly increasing healthcare spending. Between 2000 and 2004 the percentage of the working-age population covered by employer benefits fell from 68 to 63.

Unsurprisingly, lack of health insurance has been linked to poorer health results. In a study examining the health of "near elderly" adults who were not quite old enough for Medicare, the uninsured delayed medical treatments until they reached the age of Medicare eligibility. As a result, even after controlling for socio-economic factors like education, race, income, and wealth, a number of self-reported diabetes and cardiovascular health measures improved considerably for the previously uninsured once they turned 65 (McWilliams et al., 2007). This also suggests that delaying the age at which people become eligible may actually increase Medicare spending since people will enter the program with greater, and more expensive, medical needs (McWilliams et al., 2007).

Adults between 51 and 61 who were continuously uninsured were three times as likely to experience a health decline as those who were insured, even after adjustment for sociodemographic factors, medical conditions, and behavioral risk factors (Baker et al., 2001). People diagnosed with colorectal cancer who did not have insurance were 70 percent more likely than those with full insurance to die within three years (Krugman and Wells, 2006). In 2008, Oregon conducted a lottery that extended its Medicaid program to low-income individuals who did not meet the Medicaid program criteria. Almost 90,000 people applied for the lottery of 10,000 new slots, creating a natural experiment that randomly assigned individuals into insured and uninsured groups. The group that received the insurance had much higher rates of healthcare utilization and better self-reported health (Finkelstein et al., 2011).

Yet insurance does not exactly equal access. In countries that have public insurance, often not all types of services are covered. In addition, nations like Canada with public insurance often have debates about the wait that patients face for more specialized services. This is what critics of public insurance refer to as "rationing," and they argue that those with private plans have better access to healthcare. However, private insurance has its own methods of rationing. In health maintenance organizations (HMOs), sick patients have more difficulty in seeking needed care than do healthy patients (Consumer Reports, 2000). In another study, people with histories of illness like stroke or cancer had twice as much difficulty accessing medical care, even when they were insured (Himmelstein and Woolhandler, 1995). Some managed care companies also have a policy requiring pre-approval of services, even in the case of emergencies, which can restrict access to suddenly needed care.

Private insurers can also deny coverage for certain services. There are very different levels of private insurance. People often have to pay out of pocket for things like deductibles. As firms have attempted to reduce their share of rising health costs, these kinds of gaps in insurance have increased. One study defined a person as underinsured if they met one of three criteria: self-financed medical expenses were over 10 percent of income, for low-income adults medical expenses were over 5 percent of income, or deductibles equaled 5 percent of income. According to this measure, approximately 25 million people in the United States were underinsured in 2007, up 60 percent from 2003 (Schoen, Collins, and Kriss, 2008). Combining the uninsured with this measure of the underinsured, 65 million people in the United States had serious healthcare access limitations.

To make matters worse, the private system did not even deliver efficient services to those who were insured. This is the claim of proponents of the private system, who argue that competition between firms creates an efficient market, providing the best benefits at the lowest costs. But this does not appear to be the case. Although different US administrations have often attempted to unleash the efficiency of the for-profit sector, savings have stubbornly refused to follow. In 1980, Medicare attempted to create cost savings by encouraging people to sign up with private HMOs. It set the payment rate to the HMOs at 95 percent of the average costs in the public Medicare program. The assumption was that private-sector efficiency would generate a 5 percent saving. It soon became clear that the HMOs were "skimming" more healthy patients and rejecting those more prone to illnesses, who were forced back into the public program. Despite a more inherently profitable client base, the HMOs could not compete with the public plan, mostly because their administrative costs ran at 15 percent compared with Medicare's 3 percent. Patients in the HMO program cost Medicare 12 percent more than those in the traditional program (Woolhandler and Himmelstein, 2007a).

The overhead cost of administering a multi-payer system, for both reimbursing agencies and providers, is generally much larger than a single-payer public system. In the United States, this waste has been estimated at $400 billion. It is important to stress that although some of this (a healthy $10 to 15 billion) is insurance industry profit, and another portion goes into the pockets of very well-compensated chief executives, the vast majority comes from simply running the bureaucracy of private, for-profit insurance firms (Freeman, 2009). It is not only employers who are fitting the bill for this expensive insurance system. The cost of an employer-based insurance plan for a typical family of four was $19,393 in 2011, double the $9,235 in 2002 (Mayne, Girod, and Weltz, 2011: 1).

In addition to the higher bureaucratic costs of the private system, there are two other reasons that the costs of a single state insurance program would be lower despite the rhetoric of the benefits of competition. First, a single payer can put more pressure on suppliers to reduce costs. Second, private insurance companies are not cost minimizers, but profit maximizers. As a result, actions that increase costs but also increase profits will be undertaken. Private insurers can increase profits by spending money on things like marketing and risk estimation to set differential premiums. Neither of these costs needs to be incurred in a public system.

Although there has been much fearmongering about the ability of government-funded Medicare to survive, its costs have been better controlled than those in the private sector. Between 1969 and 2009 inflation-adjusted costs have escalated by 400 percent per beneficiary under Medicare, but private health insurance premiums have increased by 700 percent during the same period (Krugman, 2011a: A23). According to the Congressional Budget Office (CBO), the strictly government version of Medicare is 11 percent less expensive than private insurance (CBO , 2011a).

Private, for-profit insurance is more expensive than the public alternative, raising questions about its superior efficiency. As for the quality of service to its customers, when Joseph Newhouse, a professor of health policy at Harvard University and board member of private insurer Aetna, was interviewed in the *New York Times* about whether the US insurance industry had improved its quality of service or cost control, his answer was not convincing: "It's just very difficult to give much of an evidence-based answer to those questions ... in either direction" (Hilzenrath, 2009).

For-profit hospitals and healthcare services

Like the for-profit insurance industry, for-profit healthcare delivery is also touted as being more efficient than public ownership. However, again, empirical support for this claim is difficult to come by. Like health insurance, healthcare delivery is profit-maximizing, not cost-minimizing, and there are reasons to believe that incentives within the industry are likely to result in profit-maximizing decisions that will increase the costs of healthcare without marked improvements in health outcomes. After all, revenues in the health industry, whether they go to drug companies, doctors, or hospitals, stem from selling healthcare services, not economizing on care. Medical technology firms make money by selling expensive machines to hospitals. Drug companies earn revenue by convincing doctors to prescribe their medication. Even doctors on fee for service make more money by seeing more patients. This can lead to some very dubious practices.

The hospital company Columbia/HCA embellished the severity

of its patients' illnesses (Gottlieb, Eichenwald, and Barbanel, 1997), falsified Medicare payment forms, and billed several times for the same treatment (Eichenwald, 1997). Tenet hospitals also falsified records to overcharge Medicare (Pollack, 2003a), offered doctors kickbacks for referrals (Pollack, 2003b), and performed cardiac procedures on patients who did not need them (Eichenwald, 2003). These are examples of inethical and illegal activities. Yet the incentives in for-profit medical services are to provide as much profitable service as possible. This does not align well with a societal goal to reduce medical costs while providing quality care.

Doctors play an important role in determining how much the medical system is used. There is considerable evidence that "entrepreneurial" physicians can harm the efficiency of the healthcare system by increasing use without improving outcomes. One famous study compared the efficiency of healthcare in the Texas towns of El Paso and McAllen (Gawande, 2009). Both have similar costs of living and healthcare outcomes, yet Medicare spent $15,000 per patient in McAllen and $7,505 in El Paso. The hospitals in the two towns offered similar services and, according to Medicare's ranking of hospitals, in terms of quality of care the big hospitals in McAllen performed worse than those in El Paso on average. The much larger bill for patients in McAllen was caused by "across-the-board overuse of medicine."

> Between 2001 and 2005, critically ill Medicare patients received almost fifty percent more specialist visits in McAllen than in El Paso, and were two-thirds more likely to see ten or more specialists in a six-month period. In 2005 and 2006, patients in McAllen received twenty percent more abdominal ultrasounds, thirty percent more bone-density studies, sixty percent more stress tests with echocardiography, two hundred percent more nerve-conduction studies to diagnose carpal-tunnel syndrome, and five hundred and fifty percent more urine-flow studies to diagnose prostate troubles. They received one-fifth to two-thirds more gallbladder operations, knee replacements, breast biopsies, and bladder scopes. They also received two to three times as many pacemakers, implantable defibrillators, cardiac-bypass operations, carotid endarterectomies, and coronary-artery stents. And Medicare paid for five times as many home-nurse visits.
>
> (Gawande, 2009)

The author's explanation for this problem is a "culture of

entrepreneurship" in McAllen doctors that had not yet reached El Paso. In McAllen, often doctors had ownership of medical facilities to which they could refer patients. These trends have spread beyond McAllen's town limits. A Dartmouth Institute study blamed a "culture of entrepreneurship" when its authors found that, in situations in which the science is less than definitive, doctors figure out ways to increase their high-margin work and decrease their low-margin work. These discretionary decisions were partly responsible for the fact that different regions in the United States had vastly different health spending but very similar health results (Sirovich et al., 2008; see also Mulley, 2009). Another study found that when medical providers own labs and diagnostic equipment (like CT scanners) they are more likely to prescribe those services than those who have no ownership stake (Bernstein, 2009).

For-profit hospitals and other healthcare facilities do not appear to generate any real efficiencies in healthcare delivery. The fact that the United States has regions that are completely served by either for-profit or not for-profit hospitals provides an opportunity to compare the two ownership models. Medicare spending per capita (adjusted for health characteristics) in communities with for-profit hospitals ($5,172) was higher than in communities with non-profit hospitals ($4,440) in 1995. Further, between 1989 and 1995 costs increased by 29 percent in for-profit as opposed to 25 percent in the non-profit communities. For communities that switched all of their hospitals from non-profit to profit, per capita spending between 1989 and 1995 increased 50 percent more than for those that maintained non-profit ownership ($1,295 vs $866) (Silverman, Skinner, and Fischer, 1999). For-profit hospitals also charged more per discharged patient ($8,115) than non-profits ($7,490) between 1990 and 1994, in part because of much higher administrative costs per patient day (Woolhandler and Himmelstein, 1997). A study by Alan Sager and Deborah Socolar of the Boston University School of Public Health estimated that "one-half of health spending goes to clinical and administrative waste, excess prices, and theft" (2005: ii). In general, the larger the private share of healthcare financing, the more difficult it is to control healthcare expenditures (Evans, 2002).

Non-profit hospitals also appear to score higher on quality grounds. A study comparing the mortality rate of fee-for-service Medicare heart attack patients in non-profit and for-profit hospitals found that rates in the for-profit hospitals were 1.5 to 2 percentage points higher over a 30-day period. Further, facilities that converted from non-profit to profit experienced a 1.7 to 2 percentage point increase in mortality rates after the conversion (Shen, 2002). Similar results have been found comparing for-profit and non-profit dialysis facilities. A study tracking 500,000 patients for one year showed that those attending for-profit centers were "significantly more likely to die than those treated in non profit ones." If the sample was expanded to the entire US population using dialysis, the authors estimate that as many as 2,500 deaths each year may be due to treatment at profit, as opposed to non-profit facilities (Devereaux et al., 2002; see also Garg et al., 1999).

Patient surveys also fail to reveal a preference for care in for-profit systems. This is true whether comparing the United States with other nations in which for-profit firms play less of a role, or contrasting US profit and non-profit healthcare institutions. In the 1990s a Harris poll found that people in the United States report much lower satisfaction with their healthcare systems than do Canadian, Western European, and Japanese people (Isaacson, 1993). A 2005 survey of sicker adults in six wealthy nations found that, while no one country was a consistent laggard in all respects, "the US often stands out for inefficient care and errors" (Schoen et al., 2005). A massive survey of 82,583 Medicare patients in 182 health plans found that non-profit health plans scored higher than for-profit on measures of overall quality, access to care, and customer service (Landon et al., 2001).

On a more systemic level there is also little empirical evidence to suggest that high-cost healthcare delivers better health results. Jonathan Skinner and Elliot Fisher, two of the lead researchers in the Dartmouth Study, discovered tremendous differences in healthcare costs in different regions in the United States caused by different rates of healthcare utilization. Yet the authors also found that higher spending and greater use of healthcare did not result in "better health quality, access to care or health outcomes" (Skinner and Fisher, 2010). Their conclusion was that there is tremendous waste in the US system, and that if the costs in the high-cost areas could be brought down to those in the low-cost areas it would save trillions of dollars without any negative consequences on health outcomes.

In a review of some 150 studies comparing access, quality, and cost-effectiveness between the two ownership models in healthcare, 18 found that for-profit centers were better, 88 determined that non-profits were superior, and 43 concluded that there was no real difference (Vaillancourt and Linder, 2003). Interestingly, the United States has an excellent model of health provision that largely eschews private, for-profit delivery—the Veterans Health Administration (VA). This has been able to adopt information technology more successfully than private institutions, has been recommended as a model of equal treatment (Jha et al., 2001), quality care (Oliver, 2007), and cost control (Hendricks, Remler, and Prashker, 1999).

The pharmaceutical industry

The drug industry is an excellent example of how the industries in the MIC operate. The drug industry has successfully managed to

Race and healthcare

While the MIC has not served the general US population particularly well, minorities have fared even worse under the US model of private healthcare. According to the US Commission on Civil Rights, "equal treatment and equal access are not a reality for racial/ethnic minorities and women in the current climate of the health care industry. Many barriers limit both the quality of health care and utilization for these groups, including ... discrimination" (cited in Randall, 2002).

A large part of the reason for this is that minorities are much more likely to find themselves in socio-economic classes that are not well served by for-profit healthcare. Predictably, prior to the passage of Obama's Affordable Care Act (ACA) (which is discussed in much more detail later in the chapter), minorities made up a disproportionate share of the under or uninsured. This is an unfortunate but inevitable consequence of an employment-based insurance system when minorities are concentrated in jobs that are less likely to offer insurance benefits. Minorities are also live disproportionately in lower-income areas that are poorly served by healthcare facilities. Yet race also plays a role independent of class. Even when controlling for factors like insurance, income, and education, whites receive more thorough diagnostic work and better treatment than blacks. These effects are especially significant for black women (Randall, 2002).

In Chapter 4 we saw that race is an important explanatory factor in the social, environmental, and economic conditions that influence people's health. This is true because blacks are more likely to belong to the class that lives and works in conditions that are unhealthy, and because even within this class, these conditions are worse for blacks than for whites. The same could be said of the healthcare system that is tasked with the Herculean task of dealing with these negative outcomes. Blacks disproportionately belong to the class of people that receive particularly poor care under the US system, and even within this group blacks get worse treatment than whites.

lobby for a very favorable regulatory environment for its products, including large research and development (R&D) subsidies and extensive patent protection for new drugs. Each year, the United States spent $752 per person on prescription drugs, the highest level in the OECD. The second highest spending nation, France, spent only $599 (Peterson and Burton, 2007: 27). Much of this price difference can be attributed to lengthy patent protection in the United States, which gives drug companies a monopoly by prohibiting generic competitors. A study in the *New England Journal of Medicine* estimated that the savings from introducing a generic competitor to the widely advertised and top-selling prescription drug Lipitor would be around $4.5 billion a year (Jackevicius et al., 2012: 202).

The long patent protection for new drugs, and resulting high prices, are almost exclusively justified by the massive R&D costs associated with discovering and developing new pharmaceuticals. Yet, real questions could be asked about the extent of the private-sector contribution towards the development of new drugs compared with that of the public sector. US taxpayers pay for most of the research for new drugs, not the drug companies. This is especially true for basic research to discover breakthrough new drugs (Freeman, 2012). Taxes fund the entire National Institute of Health (NIH) budget for basic research, which hovers between $25 and $30 billion every year, as well as most of the training and research infrastructure that the industry draws on. Taxpayers also subsidize a good deal of corporate R&D through deductions and tax credits. According to the most objective data, from the National Science Foundation, drug companies spend just 10 percent of their domestic sales income on R&D, and only 18 percent of that on basic research. Thus, only 1.8 percent of sales (18 percent of 10 percent) income is spent on discovering breakthrough new drugs (Light and Lexchin, 2005: 958–60).

What are the drug companies doing with their revenue? A surprising amount goes into lobbying the US government. According to the Center for Responsive Politics (2011), between 1998 and 2011 the "pharmaceutical & other health products" industry spent $2.1 billion lobbying the US federal government. In this sector it is the pharmaceutical industry rather than "other health products" that is the big spender. The top four lobbyists are specific drug companies and the industry association.

Advertising was another big cost for drug companies. This is especially true in the United States, where drug companies are now allowed to advertise directly to the public. In 2000, pharmaceutical companies spent $2.5 billion in direct advertising. While this number seems astronomical, and it is the fastest-growing form of advertising, it only represents about 20 percent of the drug companies' total marketing budget (Mintzes et al., 2002). It seems as if it is more profitable for drug companies to get the state to extend patents and advertise than to innovate.

Even more damning, when new drugs are developed they often seem to be little different from those previously on the shelf. According to the National Institute for Health Care Management (NIHCM), 85 percent of the 1,035 new drug applications that received approval by the FDA in the United States from 1989 to 2000 do not provide significant improvement over currently marketed therapies (2002: 3). According to the NIHCM, brand manufacturers have flooded the market with product line extensions (known as "evergreening" in the industry) in response to perverse incentives related to changes in patent laws and advertising regulations. While the private contribution to drug R&D is overstated, the crucial role of the public sector is ignored. According to a Joint Economic Committee of Congress report, among the 21 drugs that had the most impact on therapeutic practice between 1965 and 1992, publicly funded research was instrumental to the development of 16, or 76 percent (Joint Economic Committee, 2000).

An excellent illustration of the manner in which drug companies operate is the glaucoma drug Xalatan. Xalatan generated $500 million in sales in 1999 alone for the Pharmacia company. Its price is also much higher in the US market than it is in other countries. The cost to the patient is about $1 a day, which might not seem like much to avoid blindness, but that is twice as much as a Japanese patient would pay, and places it beyond the reach of many low-income people. Pharmacia criticizes the low, regulated international prices and justifies its US rate by arguing that innovation is expensive. Yet, the scientific discovery behind the drug was not made at Pharmacia, but at Columbia University by Hungarian science professor Laszlo Bito, who had received $4 million in funding from the NIH. Pharmacia actually purchased the rights to the drug for between $100,000 and $150,000. Pharmacia then spent tens of millions of dollars developing the product so that it was safer, and guiding it through the expensive clinical trial process to bring Xalatan to market. Yet the big expense for Pharmacia is marketing. In 1999, 40 percent of the company's revenue went to marketing and administration. The entire R&D budget was half of that. A fundamental part of its marketing campaign is to persuade doctors to prescribe Xalatan, so much of its advertising goes to "detail men" who make personal calls on doctors and have given away more than a million free samples (Gerth and Stolberg, 2000: 1).

Drug companies, universities, and independent research

To a remarkable extent, then, medical centers have become supplicants to the drug companies, deferring to them in ways that would have been unthinkable even twenty years ago. Often, academic researchers are little more than hired hands who supply human subjects and collect data according to instructions from corporate paymasters. The sponsors keep the data, analyze it, write the papers, and decide whether and when and where to submit them for publication. In multi-center trials, researchers may not even be allowed to see all of the data, an obvious impediment to science and a perversion of standard practice .... Medical centers increasingly act as though meeting industry's needs is a legitimate purpose of an academic institution.

Much of the rationalization for the pervasive research connections between industry and academia rests on the Bayh–Dole Act of 1980, which has acquired the status of holy writ in academia. Bayh–Dole permits—but does not require, as many researchers claim—universities to patent discoveries that stem from government-funded research and then license them exclusively to companies in return for royalties. (Similar legislation applies to work done at the NIH itself.) In this way, academia and industry are partners, both benefiting from public support. Until Bayh–Dole, all government-funded discoveries were in the public domain.

A less-appreciated outcome of Bayh–Dole is that drug companies no longer have to do their own creative, early-stage research. They can, and increasingly do, rely on universities and start-up companies for that. In fact, the big drug companies now concentrate mainly on the late-stage development of drugs they've licensed from other sources, as well as on producing variations of top-selling drugs already on the market—called "me-too" drugs. There is very little innovative research in the modern pharmaceutical industry, despite its claims to the contrary.

Source: excerpted from Angell (2010). (For an overview of the drug industry see Angell, 2004.)

Profits in the MIC

Although the US system does not service the general public, or even large segments of the business community, particularly well, it does benefit the MIC. Doctors in the United States are better compensated than in other countries. In 2004, US general practitioners earned an average of $161,000, the highest figure in a 21-country Congressional Research Service study (see Figure 5.1).

Doctors are not the only members of the MIC that are benefiting from the current structure of the US healthcare industry. Out of 51 industries analyzed in the Fortune 500, three of the fifteen most profitable industries belong to the MIC (see Table 5.2). Although the insurance industry faced a bit of a down year in 2008, it bounced back in 2009, increasing profits by 56 percent to a record $12.2 billion (Walker, 2010). The drug industry is very profitable. Johnson & Johnson alone made a profit of $13 billion in 2008, making it the ninth most profitable company on the Fortune 500. The big drug companies consistently have profits three to five times greater than most Fortune 500 companies. In 2002, the combined profits of the ten drug companies in the Fortune 500 equaled half the combined profits of all the other 490 major corporations (Light and Lexchin, 2005: 958–60). In 2008, the pharmaceutical industry was the third most profitable industry in the United States (behind

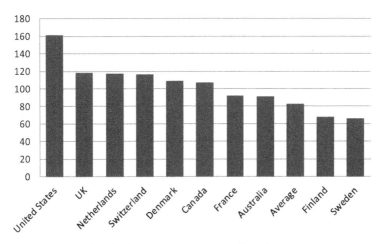

Figure 5.1 General medical practitioners' pay in selected countries
(in $1,000s)

Source: Peterson and Burton (2007).

Table 5.2 Profit rank of the top 3 MIC industries (out of 51 industries in the United States)

		Pharmaceuticals	Medical products	Ins: life, health (stock)
2005	Rank	5	6	12
	Profits %	15.7	13.2	10.3
2006	Rank	2	6	12
	Profits %	19.6	13.5	10.7
2007	Rank	3	4	9
	Profits %	15.8	15.2	10.6
2008	Rank	3	4	22
	Profits %	19.3	16.3	4.6

Note: The ranking is by profits as a percentage of revenue.

Source: *Fortune* (2009).

communications equipment and internet services), with profits a very healthy 19 percent of revenues according to the Fortune 500 (Fortune, 2009). Medical products were not far behind with profits making up 16.3 percent of revenues. The highest total profit in the industry was the $2.2 billion earned by Medtronic. Although 2008 was a down year for the insurance industry, MetLife still managed to turn a $3.2 billion profit (Fortune, 2009). The tremendous profitability of these industries creates both the motive and the wherewithal to influence healthcare policy in the United States.

ECONOMICS IN SUPPORT OF THE MIC

The U.S. experience has shown that private markets and commercial competition have made things worse, not better, for our healthcare system. That could have been predicted, because healthcare is clearly a public concern and a personal right of all citizens. By its very nature, it is fundamentally different from most other goods and services distributed in commercial markets. Markets simply are not designed to deal effectively with the delivery of medical care—which is a social function that needs to be addressed in the public sector.

(Dr. Arnold Relman, professor emeritus at the Harvard Medical School, testifying before the Senate of Canada, in Canadian Health Coalition letter to Barack Obama, May 7, 2009).

Proponents of a private healthcare system can draw from a long list of academic economists who argue for the superiority of the private market approach to health. At the core of these justifications is that medical services are essentially no different from any other commodity, from houses to clothing, and that the same market system that delivers a nice home can also deliver low-cost, reliable healthcare. Setting aside, for the moment, the problems with this claim even in the market for housing, there are reasons to believe that healthcare is different in many crucial respects from other, more conventional markets.

The hallmark of what health economist Robert Evans calls the "naïve" economic model, is that prices and output for healthcare services are efficiently arrived at through the interaction of consumer demand and producer supply (Evans, 1984: 23). Consumers will obtain healthcare if the marginal benefit of improved health exceeds the marginal cost of obtaining that care. The benefits of healthcare treatment depend on individual preferences for good health. Suppliers will provide care if the marginal revenue exceeds the marginal cost of provision. In this model, an "efficient" level of care is provided and consumed that reflects the preferences of consumers and the cost of healthcare. If the market can deliver an efficient level of care, then any intervention in the market will be an unwelcome development.

For example, if public health insurance provides free healthcare (as is the case for many health services in Canada), this model would conclude that reducing the cost of a visit to the doctor (it would not fall to zero because there is still a cost for people's time) will lead to people overusing medical care since they will demand care for which they have a lower marginal benefit. It will also lead to wait times since the demand for services will likely exceed supply. This will disadvantage those whose time has a higher value, like high-wage earners, since they will be less willing to tolerate the queues that result from the excess demand for health services. The recommendations that follow from this model are to ensure competition in the supply of healthcare, greater reliance on prices, and a reduction in the role of publicly funded insurance so that patients bear more of the cost (see for example Epstein, 1997).

One of the most influential studies in this vein was Michael Grossman's (1972) article on the demand for healthcare. Grossman borrowed from the economics of human capital formation to argue that people invest in their own health in much the same way that people invest in education. People start off with a stock of health that deteriorates, at an increasing rate, over time. Investments in healthcare are both a consumption good and an investment that improves people's future health to reduce the number of days spent in unproductive sickness. People make optimizing decisions on how much to invest in health based on the costs and benefits. The Grossman model predicts how health demand will be impacted by a number of factors, like the prices of medical care and changes in income. For example, an individual's wage will influence how much medical care they demand in two ways. On one hand, a higher wage makes medical care more costly because the time that it takes to make investments in health (doctor's appointments or trips to the gym) is more valuable. On the other hand, "the higher a person's wage rate the greater value to him of an increase in healthy time" (Grossman, 1972: 242). Overall the second impact should outweigh the first, leading to an increased demand for health as wages rise.

This kind of modeling of healthcare has more academic influence in the United States than elsewhere. The WHO international comparison of textbooks of health economics pointed out that the three dominant US textbooks used a market-oriented approach in which individual utility maximization was the principal behavioral assumption, and the "special features of health care are treated as variations on the perfectly competitive model" (Hersh-Cochran, 1989: 214). This is remarkably different from a Canadian text by Evans that is a "clear critique of the neoclassical approach" (Hersh-Cochran, 1989: 214).

The Grossman model supports the conclusions of efficiency in the private healthcare market. In this model, healthcare consumers are able to judge their medical needs accurately in order select the optimal amount of care given their preferences and constraints. Yet there are some vital problems with assuming that healthcare can be analyzed like any other market. Perhaps most fundamentally, we might object to the implications of Grossman's model that people with higher incomes will receive more medical care and live more healthy lives. In fact, the egalitarian idea that healthcare should not be dependent on income lies behind the commitment to universal healthcare in countries other than the United States. The right to healthcare is even enshrined in the Universal Declaration of Human Rights (1948). However, even if an egalitarian claim to healthcare access for all is not persuasive, there are also efficiency reasons to question applying regular market principles to healthcare.

Given that the actual costs of many health procedures are greatly in excess of what any family could reasonably be expected to pay from their own savings, insurance is a common feature of this market. Some health analysts have argued that the main problem with insurance, not only in health but also in any market, is that it creates the problem of moral hazard (Pauly, 1968). This means that people who are insured will change their behavior to take fewer precautions, making them more likely to use their insurance. In healthcare this would mean that those who are insured overuse the system because they take fewer actions to prevent themselves from having to use healthcare, and because the costs of health services are not fully borne by the patients, so they consume services whose benefit to them is less than the cost of provision. So theorists in the moral hazard tradition argue that insurance creates risky and wasteful behavior by those insured (Gladwell, 2005). If this theory is correct, then universal public insurance should lead to an overwhelming increase in demand for healthcare. According to John Nyman (2003) of the University of Minnesota, the sway that this theory holds over US health economists explains their lack of support for most programs that would expand insurance coverage.

It also, logically, supports an increase in what has euphemistically been called a "consumer-directed" approach to health (for example Cogan, Hubbard, and Kessler, 2006). What consumer-directed in fact means is that the consumer should be responsible for a greater proportion of the medical bill. So the move toward higher deductibles and co-payments in the United States should not merely be interpreted as an effort to offload health costs by firms and insurance companies, but as a move to making the healthcare system more efficient by having consumers put their money where their health is (Gladwell, 2005).

Economists concerned about moral hazard argue that the efficiency of the healthcare system will be improved by ending the tax subsidy for employer-based insurance and increasing co-insurance payments by as much as 67 percent (Feldstein, 1973; see also Manning and Marquis, 1996). Again, these claims are only reasonable if the consumers of healthcare can accurately assess the benefits that they receive from healthcare. If they cannot do so, then the most likely outcome of these policies is that people will reduce the use of healthcare but will be unable to discern desirable economies from capricious ones—a point to which we will return.

The other problem with insurance is known as adverse selection. The idea behind adverse selection is that insurance attracts customers who are more likely to claim. If insurance companies set fees according to the amount that they are likely to spend on healthcare for the average person, then individuals in good health and unlikely to require medical care will not purchase insurance. Those more prone to illness, on the other hand, will find insurance an attractive proposition. Insurance companies will then be burdened with high-cost customers and an unprofitable business. This becomes a vicious cycle: if the insurance companies raise their rates as a result, they will only then be attractive to an even less healthy customer base, and so on.

One way around this problem is to pool people together in large groups and force them to pay for insurance, even though this inevitably means that the healthy subsidize the sick. In the United States, this was achieved with a certain amount of success by large employers providing insurance since they could be assumed to have a sufficiently large pool of workers that the adverse selection problem would not be an issue. However, because of the dramatically escalating costs of healthcare, workers who have health problems are drawn to those companies that still offer a solid health benefits package. According to the chairman of Starbucks, Howard Schultz, "what's perverse is that companies like ours who are doing the right thing are actually paying more" (Picard, 2005). In an effort to stem this tide, employers are using the health of potential recruits as hiring criteria. The *New York Times* reported that Wal-Mart suggested that the addition of physical tasks to otherwise non-physical labor could weed out applicants with health problems (Krugman and Wells, 2006). The most obvious solution to the adverse selection problem is to ensure that everyone takes out insurance. This is part of the logic behind universal public systems. The United States has attempted to replicate at least the universal aspect of this in Obama's healthcare plan by forcing everyone not insured under one of the government programs to purchase private insurance.

It is not only insurance that makes healthcare an atypical market. It is also characterized by profound uncertainty for the consumer. Information asymmetry is the term economists use to describe a market in which one party in an exchange is much better informed than the other. The pioneering work in the area used the market for second-hand automobiles as its example (Akerloff, 1970). While the asymmetry problems exist in many markets, the information problem is greater in healthcare than in most other markets for a number of reasons. First, patients often face greater uncertainty about healthcare than would exist for other products. While it is relatively easy to conduct research on the automobile market to reduce the information asymmetry, it is more difficult for medical consumers to read up on the latest medical techniques or scientific advances. This problem is exacerbated because often medical interventions can have different impacts on different individuals. Second, the consequences of making a bad decision in healthcare are much more serious than in other markets, making consumers much less likely to go against their physician's advice. Finally, doctors act as gatekeepers into medical care, which restricts consumers' ability to act independently from their physicians (see the box on page 158).

Evidence does suggest that people have difficulty discerning necessary from unnecessary consumption of healthcare. A famous study by the Rand Corporation in the 1970s randomly assigned US families to health plans that required them to pay zero, 25, 50, or 95 percent of their medical expenses. The "consumer-driven" model would predict two things. First, those families who pay less of the direct cost of their treatment will consume more than those who pay a higher percentage. Second, the higher-percentage families will make more efficient medical choices. The Rand study found that only the first of these predictions came true. While families with higher payments did take up fewer medical treatments, they used less of all kinds of services, even those that would have been extremely valuable. Poorer families, predictably, were more negatively impacted by higher payments and cut back on medical care that could have led to substantial health benefits. For example, people on lower incomes with high blood pressure showed a greater improvement in the free plan, resulting in a mortality improvement of 10 percent (Newhouse, 1993: 339).

Decisions on healthcare options are not made primarily by consumers; rather, they are made by consumers on the advice of their doctor—what economists call the agency relationship. For most patients this advice has a strong enough weight that "doctor's orders" actually has some meaning. If the doctor could somehow fully understand the condition of the patient—their preferences, their desires, and their life circumstances—then it might be possible to claim that the advice of the doctor is the same as the wishes of the patient, but this symbiosis is difficult to achieve. Even if it were possible, a doctor's advice might not represent their patient's desires if they have differing interests, which is often the case. This is especially true since the United States has refused to follow the advice of the former editor of the *New England Journal of Medicine*,

Arnold Relman, who argued that doctors should not be able to gain financially from any part of the healthcare system except directly from their own services (Relman, 1980). The fact that physicians are both expert advisers on what is necessary and suppliers of those services gives rise to the possibility of supply-induced demand (SID). On the one hand doctors are their patients' agents with respect to healthcare, while on another they have their own interests, which include income and status in their profession.

SID occurs when the physicians/suppliers of services can influence demand. Intuitively, this would appear to be the case in healthcare, and empirical evidence suggests that it is common. This is the most logical reason for the fact that high-cost and high-utilization medical systems have failed to produce superior healthcare results. Studies have shown that when doctors own medical facilities like labs or technology like magnetic resonance imaging (MRI) machines, they prescribe their own services more often than doctors who do not have an ownership stake (Bernstein, 2009). Studies have also found that an increase in physicians in a region result in an increase in per capita utilization and an increase in prices, which is the opposite of what the economic model would predict without SID. Some

Doctors as gatekeepers for the MIC

Every dollar that physicians earn for themselves is only a fraction of their effect on the overall demand for health care services. As gatekeepers they control patient use of much of the rest of the medical system, including technology, pharmaceuticals, specialists, nursing and hospital visits. In the less regulated market and profit oriented US health care system dominated by the MIC the effects of SID can be substantial. A survey of hospital Chief Financial Officers by the Healthcare Financial Management Association (HFMA) found that physicians generated an average of $1.54 million per year for their hospitals. The most lucrative specialization for the hospital was neurosurgery, in which doctors created an average of $2.8 million. Invasive cardiologists ($2.2 million a year), orthopedic surgeons ($2.1 million a year), and general surgeons ($2.1 million a year) also ranked above the average. Surgeons are not the only big revenue generators. General internists generate $1.7 million a year, and family physicians $1.6 million each year.

(Commins, 2010).

surgeries like appendectomies are particularly susceptible to SID, since patients are particularly unable to determine whether the procedure is necessary, and it has no long-term detrimental impact on the patient. The research on this subject has consistently shown a relationship between the type of physician payment and the number of surgeries performed. In one study, the rate of surgery was 78 percent higher when doctors were paid through fee for service rather than by capitation (fee per patient) despite similar patient characteristics (Shafrin, 2010; see also Hemenway et al., 1990; Hillman, Pauly, and Kerstein, 1989).

The "naïve" economic model in which supply and demand interact to produce efficient outcomes provides an important intellectual justification for a private, for-profit, market-driven healthcare system. However this is not a particularly realistic description of the healthcare market, and it is one that is not given much intellectual weight outside the United States. Insurance creates problems of moral hazard and adverse selection. Further, the fundamental uncertainty that surrounds how any healthcare treatment translates into good health casts considerable doubt on the idea of consumer sovereignty in this market. Rather it is doctors, as imperfect agents for their patients, who drive demand in healthcare. A more realistic understanding of the nature of healthcare calls into question the efficiency claims made by proponents of a market-based approach. The economists who provide the intellectual justification for a market-oriented consumer-driven healthcare system fit well with the needs of MIC. As we shall see in the next chapter, an analysis of healthcare rooted in SID lends itself to a very different policy perspective.

SID: physicians and the drug industry

It is difficult for consumers to judge their own needs in the area of prescription drugs. If a person is told that they require a certain medication to alleviate an illness, few are comfortable enough in their knowledge of pharmacology to second-guess their doctor. Patients are also not permitted to wander down to the local drug store and pick up a few pills without a prescription. The physician's gatekeeper role places them in a position from which they can have a strong influence on the demand for drugs. Realizing this, drug companies have worked hard to cultivate relationships with doctors in a variety of creative ways. Psychiatrist Daniel Carlat and his wife enjoyed an all-expenses-paid "training" weekend in New York, including a Broadway show, after he agreed to talk to fellow physicians about the antidepressant drug Effexor. He was paid $750 per "lunch and learn" session, in which he gave a ten-minute lecture on the benefits of the Effexor to other doctors (Jack, 2011).

These kinds of perks and payments from drug companies to doctors are routine practice in the industry. Abbott Laboratories was chastized by the British Pharmaceutical Industry in 2006 when its sales reps entertained doctors at greyhound races, Wimbledon, and a lap-dancing club. Eight different drug companies paid a combined $320 million to 18,000 doctors. Some were particularly well compensated. The top ten recipients pocketed a minimum of $250,000 each. The head of Sanofi-Aventis defended the physician–drug company relationship with the claim that "doctors are professionals and I have every confidence in their judgment," so payments should have no impact on their professional integrity (Jack, 2011). If doctors' decisions were actually unaffected by drug company persuasion, we would have to question why drug companies keep spending so much money on them. It is physicians' ability to induce demand for drugs through the power of the prescription that creates the incentive for drug companies to offer perks to doctors.

PREDICTABLE: OBAMA'S HEALTHCARE PLAN

I see no reason why the United States of America, the wealthiest country in the history of the world, spending 14 percent of its gross national product on health care, cannot provide basic health insurance to everybody. And that's what Jim is talking about when he says everybody in, nobody out—a single-payer health care plan, a universal health care plan. That's what I'd like to see. But as all of you know, we may not get there immediately. Because first we've got to take back the White House, we've got to take back the Senate, and we've got to take back the House.

(Barack Obama in 2003)

By 2008 the Senate and House were Democratic and Obama was president.

The fact that President Obama chose to reduce the number of uninsured through the complicated, privately led, Affordable Care Act (ACA) rather than a public scheme reflects a compromise between the strength of the MIC and the groundswell of discontent with US healthcare. A Canadian-style public single insurer was never seriously considered, although as we shall see in Chapter 6, this might have been an obvious solution. Indeed, a proposal by a small group of Democrats to create a public insurer that would compete with private industry (a discarded plank in the Obama presidential campaign of 2008) died a rapid death facing opposition from Republicans, the insurance industry, and conservative Democrats (Marmor and Oberlander, 2010: 2). As we highlighted earlier in the chapter, business and the MIC are much more powerful politically in the United States than those bodies that represent low-waged workers and the other uninsured people (Sparer, 2009).

The starting assumption of the Obama Administration was that universal coverage would never be achieved if it were opposed by the political and financial clout of the MIC, so a proposal had to be crafted from which the MIC would benefit. This might explain why the ACA has focused on expanding coverage in a manner that, although it constrains private insurance companies in some ways, improves their revenue base by expanding the number of people who will take out private insurance and rules out any public option. It also explains why cost control measures are fairly weak. After all, one dollar of healthcare spending is one dollar of MIC income, so controlling costs necessarily means constraining corporate revenue and can be expected to meet MIC opposition. One of the lessons taken from Clinton's failed healthcare reform of 1994, which did contain more structural constraints on costs, was that no reform was likely to succeed that was strongly opposed by the medical industry (Marmor, Oberlander, and White, 2009: 486).

A more cynical interpretation of Obama's political calculus in healthcare is that he was not free of MIC influence. His election benefited from $19.5 million from the healthcare industries, far more than the $7.4 million given to his Republican opponent John McCain. This may be a small fraction of the $750 million that Obama raised overall, but firms do not spend millions without hoping to benefit in some manner. Of course, Obama was not alone in receiving funding from the MIC between the formulation and passage of the ACA. Max Baucus, chairman of the Senate Finance Committee (which drafted the Senate's healthcare legislation) received $2 million between 2005 and 2010 from the healthcare sector. In return, he met 20 times with representatives of the MIC in 2009, while public interest groups were granted only 12 meetings with him. In all, the MIC donated $28 million to various politicians in 2009–10 (Tomasky, 2010: 14).

Lobbying activity by the MIC also spiked during the debate about healthcare reform. At its apex in 2009, for every single member of the House and Senate there were six healthcare lobbyists, some 3,300 in all. The 25 highest-spending organizations in healthcare lobbying spent a combined $288 million in 2009. One of the strongest opponents of healthcare reform, the US Chamber of Commerce, spent $71 million in the last quarter of 2009 alone. PhRMA, the largest drug lobbyist, spent $26 million. This money did appear to pay some dividends. Until doctors, nurses, and medical students supporting public insurance threatened a public demonstration at the White House Health Care Summit, it did not contain a single participant advocating a single-payer, universal system to provide a counterpoint to the tide of MIC opinion (Bernstein, 2009). Lobbying on healthcare is not left to outsiders. When Baucus met with healthcare representatives, two of the lobbyists in the meeting were former chiefs of his staff, David Castagnetti and Jeffrey Forbes. Of the 165 people that PhRMA employed to lobby for its various interests, 137 have had government experience (Tomasky, 2010: 12). Of course, lobbying was done by those who supported healthcare reform as well. The American Association of Retired People (AARP), which favors expanding coverage, even when it was proposed that some of the money for this would come from cuts to Medicare, spent $21 million in 2009. The AFL-CIO contributed a much more modest $2 million lobbying in support of healthcare reform (Tomasky, 2010: 12).

The MIC also financed advertisements to influence public opinion. Six large insurance companies pooled between $10 and $20 million for television ads opposing meaningful healthcare reform that might damage the industry. In the end, the provisions in the ACA were sufficiently favorable to pharmaceutical companies that PhRMA spent $100 million on ads that supported Obama's reforms (Tomasky, 2010: 12). This simultaneously highlights how Obama chose to craft reform that would benefit the MIC and how its influence dramatically reduced the likelihood of any but the most marginal changes to the US healthcare system.

Even so, the largely MIC-friendly ACA was too much reform for many. No Republicans voted for the bill because it increased health costs to many businesses, taxed "Cadillac" insurance, and increased government healthcare subsidies. They framed the modest ACA reforms as a "government takeover" of medicine that would result in "death panels" and "pulling the plug on grandma" (Marmor and Oberlander, 2010: 1). A more radical restructuring of the industry, involving a more meaningful role for government, would have attracted even stronger opposition from Republicans and alienated many Democrats. The opponents of the ACA went so far as to launch an unsuccessful challenge to its constitutionality before the conservative United States Supreme Court.

After a predictably epic political struggle, the US government passed the ACA in 2010. It was backed by President Obama to control the very high US healthcare spending and provide insurance for more people. Its final provisions were a bit complicated, to put it mildly, but the rudiments of the bill were that the first goal would be addressed through some cost-containment measures in the government-funded programs, and the second would be addressed by forcing all of those not eligible for Medicare or Medicaid to purchase private insurance. In exchange for the emphasis on private insurance in the Obama reform, insurance companies would face some restrictions on their operations.

More people were insured by expanding Medicaid and making private insurance more easily available. All those who earned less than 133 percent of the federal poverty level were eligible for Medicaid. Further, income became the only criterion for coverage, rather than the previous exclusion of single adults without children. The ACA also filled in the so-called "donut-hole" in prescription drug coverage under Medicare. Under the previous provisions, people were responsible for costs between a low threshold and a much higher level of spending. Under the ACA, this gap was eliminated. Those who did not qualify for Medicaid, did not have employer-based plans, and had incomes below 400 percent of the poverty level, would purchase subsidized private insurance on health benefit "exchanges" set up and run at either the state or federal level. Individuals were "forced" to buy insurance in the sense that they would face a tax penalty of $95 per person or 1 percent of taxable income (whichever is greater) starting in 2014 if they refused to purchase insurance. This penalty increased fairly rapidly, so that by 2016 it would be the greater of $695 or 2.5 percent of taxable income (Marmor and Oberlander, 2010: 3). Since some people would opt to pay the penalty rather than purchase insurance, some of the population was expected to remain uninsured. Forcing people to purchase insurance was not simply a political attempt to swell the revenues of insurance companies (although it did coincidentally do this). It was also designed to solve the problem of adverse selection by pooling people into exchanges.

There was also a range of provisions to encourage firms to offer insurance to their workforce. The specific provisions differed depending on the size of the firm. Firms with under 50 employees received tax credits if they provided coverage for their employees, but were not required to provide employer-based health insurance. Firms with over 50 employees that did not offer health insurance were penalized. The penalty for these firms provided a good illustration of the complexity of the ACA provisions:

> If an employer does offer insurance to its workers but at least one full-time employee obtains coverage through the exchange with a subsidy, the employer will be assessed $3,000 for each employee getting a subsidy or $2,000 per full-time employee, whichever is less.
> (Blumberg, 2010: 2)

Firms with over 100 employees also had to offer health insurance, but almost all of them did so already. There was to be some extra costs to these firms, however, since a greater number of workers at large companies were likely to take up coverage given the penalties for not doing so. Employees of firms, mostly in the under-50-worker category, that did not provide insurance would have to use the exchanges or pay the fine for not doing so.

In exchange for creating incentives to purchase private insurance, the insurance industry would face increased regulation, prohibiting its most odious previous practices. Insurance companies were prevented from dropping people when they became ill. They were not able to refuse coverage or charge higher rates to those with existing conditions. They were obliged to keep young adults on their parents' plan until they reach 26 (many had previously dropped them at 19). Lifetime coverage limits were prohibited and there were restrictions on annual limits. Finally, insurance companies had to spend a fixed percentage of their income on direct health-related spending. Ending these practices would improve people's experience with health insurance coverage, but if past history on healthcare regulation (or any industry regulation) in the United States has taught any lesson, it is that when rules jeopardize profits, firms will find inventive ways to circumvent them. As a result, the extent to which these new regulations will actually change insurance company behavior has yet to be determined.

There is very little in the ACA that addressed the chronic issue of rising healthcare costs. Within the Medicare system, the ACA legislated a reduction in spending increases by limiting payments to hospitals and private insurers. Outside Medicare, the cost-containment measures were more limited. As mentioned previously, private insurers faced a limit on how much revenue could be spent on non-medical costs. In addition, a "Cadillac tax" was imposed on the most expansive, and expensive, health insurance plans. The hope was that this would cut the number of high-end plans that supposedly offered "luxury" care with benefits often of low value. This was obviously a controversial method of cutting costs, and in any case was not slated for introduction until 2018, creating some uncertainty about whether it would be implemented by a future president (Marmor and Oberlander, 2010: 5). All of these stopgap measures were made necessary by the refusal of the ACA to take a more systemic approach to cutting costs. Other wealthy countries spend much less than the United States, primarily because the government has a much broader role. This permits the state to set targets for health spending and regulate payments to healthcare providers (Marmor and Oberlander, 2010: 6).

The ACA contained some positive changes to US healthcare. The greatest accomplishment of the ACA was that it expanded health insurance to many previously uncovered people. The number of non-elderly adults without insurance would decrease by 28 million. Further, the greatest declines in the uninsured would be among those at the lower end of the income spectrum. Of the total of 28 million, 19 million of those who stood to gain insurance had incomes below 200 percent of the federal poverty level (Buettgens, Garrett, and Holahan, 2010).

Yet many of the previous problems remained. Many of the insured still faced discouragingly high costs that limited their use of healthcare. Indeed, some people remained uninsured either because the subsidized insurance was still too expensive (but they were not eligible for Medicaid) or they were sufficiently confident in their continued rude health that they would opt to pay the penalty rather than purchase insurance (Marmor and Oberlander, 2010: 4). In addition, the problems related to tying insurance to employment still remained, as both a growing cost for firms and a disincentive for workers to leave jobs with good insurance plans.

The ACA was also predicted to save the government some money. The CBO was asked to review the fiscal impact of the ACA when the Republicans in the House proposed its elimination with the inflammatorily named Repealing the Job-Killing Health Care Law

Act, and estimated that the ACA would reduce federal deficits by $143 billion between 2010 and 2019. Although the ACA was predicted to increase spending by $788 billion on things like increased Medicaid coverage and subsidies for employer insurance, it was also predicted to reduce spending on Medicare and generate revenue primarily through increasing the Hospital Insurance Payroll Tax and fees on manufacturers and insurance companies (CBO, 2011b: 4; Krugman, 2011b: A23). However, even should these projected savings have come to pass (and the experience of Massachusetts outlined below suggests that they might not), the ACA could best be described as working at the margins of healthcare spending rather than getting to the core problems. The ACA did not address the problematic incentives in the healthcare industry that lead profit-driven firms to oversupply their services. As a result, even if costs to the government were to decline, costs to households and businesses would likely continue to escalate.

While the passage of the ACA is too recent for any analysis beyond educated forecasting, it is possible to draw on one state-level precedent. The ACA was modeled on the 2006 Massachusetts healthcare reform passed when Mitt Romney was governor. Many of the provisions were certainly similar. Massachusetts expanded the number of people insured through a combination of broader state coverage and the carrot/stick approach to private insurance. It contained penalties for individuals and firms that did not obtain coverage as well as subsidies for low-income individuals who opted for private insurance. As was forecast for the ACA, although the Massachusetts plan did reduce the number of uninsured in the state by somewhere between 60 and 80 percent, it fell short of universal coverage (Nardin, Himmelstein, and Woolhandler, 2009: 6).

Yet, the experience of the Massachusetts model should give people some cause for concern. Healthcare costs to households have risen. Many lower-income residents, who received free care under the old state plan, faced payments of various forms under the new system, deterring them from seeking needed medical care. A middle-income individual on the cheapest plan could pay almost $10,000 for premiums, deductibles, and co-insurance if they got sick (Nardin et al., 2009: 8). It has also been more expensive for the state than originally predicted, with costs rising from $1.1 billion in 2008 to a forecast $1.3 billion in 2009 (Nardin et al., 2009: 5). As with the Obama plan, Massachusetts created another layer in the administrative apparatus of healthcare with its state-led exchange (called the Connector), which has added an extra 4 to 5 percentage points to the administrative overhead cost of private insurance (Nardin et al., 2009: 13). More generally, the Massachusetts plan did nothing to solve the basic cost driver, which is the overuse of high-cost care at the expense of cheaper, more effective primary care. Finally, those with direct experience with the new program were not particularly impressed. A survey of people who were affected by the new legislation found that 44 percent believed that new plan hurt the uninsured (who did receive some level of care prior to the new plan because the state provided funds to hospitals that treated the uninsured) while only 35 percent believed that the reform had helped. Of those affected by the reform, half said they had been made worse off (Nardin et al., 2009: 10).

The MIC, however, fared well under the Massachusetts plan. Rate increases made for record profits at large hospitals like Massachusetts General. Insurance companies, which lobbied hard for the plan, had hundreds of thousands of new customers (Woolhandler and Himmelstein, 2007b).

These trends were especially worrying since Massachusetts was starting from a relatively advantageous position in terms of its healthcare record. The number of uninsured under the old system was 10 percent in 2006, considerably lower than the national average. It was also a relatively wealthy state, with a healthier tax base than most in the country (Nardin et al., 2009: 3). The nation as a whole should have been concerned about the modest benefits achieved under favorable conditions in Massachusetts.

The limited success of the Massachusetts plan may partly explain why the ACA was not particularly popular with the US public. A 2010 survey by the Kaiser Family Foundation found that 48 percent supported the bill and 41 percent were opposed—and this was one of the more positive polls. Further, a substantial 42 percent of those surveyed admitted that they were confused about just what provisions were in the ACA (Marmor and Oberlander, 2010: 1). The obvious question is why Obama would opt for an unpopular, complicated grab bag of policies that did not provide universal access or meaningfully address cost escalation. The short answer is that the ACA reflected the same political and economic powers that shaped US healthcare policy over the longer term, which meant that the obvious solution of more direct state influence and a public, single-payer insurance system was not seriously considered.

Obama swept to power with a promise of change. Yet the shortcomings of the ACA were the inevitable result of attempting to improve healthcare coverage without changing the broader class forces that have shaped the US political economy over the last 30 years. A particularly powerful and well-entrenched subsection of the business community was able to ensure that the genuine dissatisfaction with US healthcare was channeled into legislation that it found largely very acceptable. The less politically powerful broader populace fared less well. Healthcare coverage was expanded under the ACA, but only by relying on increasingly expensive private plans. The unsatisfying compromise that was the ACA was yet further proof that the current alignment of US political and economic forces creates huge obstacles for any progressive legislation. No sweeping progressive legislation has been passed for over three decades, and the ACA certainly did not reverse that trend.

CONCLUSION

The unique US healthcare system is not a result of any genuine expression of the will of the people. Rather, its emphasis on market-driven, for-profit delivery of insurance and services is the result of conflict in society between very different healthcare interests. Evidence from both other countries and within the United States suggests that costs could be lowered and access improved without any sacrifice of medical outcomes. The population in general would benefit in terms of both access and efficiency from a healthcare system with more government intervention. Even many businesses are ambivalent about the corporate-centered model currently in place in the United States because of its impact on their health costs. Yet the MIC has been able to maintain, and in many cases expand, its role in the US system despite evidence of its harmful effects. This can only be explained by examining the way businesses, in general, and the MIC in particular, wield power in the US political and economic system.

In making the intellectual case for a market-driven healthcare system that is amenable to health industry interests, the MIC has been able to draw on the work of some leading health economists. Their consumer-driven medical model suggests that a for-profit, market model will deliver the socially optimal level of healthcare, just as is the case in any other market. While there are reasons to doubt efficiency claims in many markets, the healthcare market is perhaps one of the ones in which it most obviously fails. Beyond the moral question about making access to medical care dependent on income, there are structural features of the market for health that violate the assumptions of the usual economic demand and supply model. The issue of insurance raises problems of moral hazard and adverse selection. More importantly perhaps, the assumption that healthcare consumers are usually in a position to judge their medical needs is heroic. More realistically, it is medical professionals, not patients, who drive demand, creating SID. Adding these more realistic elements into the economics of healthcare demolishes the efficiency claims of a for-profit, market-driven healthcare model, and is precisely the reason that all other developed countries have opted for substantial state intervention.

Obama's ACA was the latest example of how the conflict between different groups in society over US healthcare has so often played out. The US population would benefit from expanding access and lowering costs. The fact that access was improved should not be downplayed. Millions who were previously without health insurance were insured. Yet, this was done in a manner that was very favorable to the MIC. A single-payer public system, and even a public competitor to private insurance, was never seriously considered because of the perceived impossibility of passing any reform that went so strongly against the interests of the MIC, even when it was the obvious solution to the twin problems of access and cost escalation. Further, private insurers were guaranteed a host of new clients under the new mandatory rules.

A dramatic restructuring of the US healthcare system, not the tinkering reforms of the ACA, is required if the United States is to genuinely improve its medical system. The power of the MIC as a well-positioned faction of the business community creates a substantial impediment to the realization of this goal—just as Relman predicted it would in 1980. Yet history also suggests that it would not be impossible. Previous progressive legislation faced similarly staunch opposition from business, yet more concerted efforts by more organized movements meant that they were successful. Similarly, the reason that other countries have more favorable social legislation, including better healthcare, is that they have been better able to turn social demands into political results. The final chapter highlights a few examples of the successes that have been achieved in other countries.

6

THREE EASY LESSONS

Countries and regions where economic resources (such as income and employment) and social resources (such as health care, education and family supportive services) are better distributed have better health indicators.

(Navarro et al., 2004: 222)

People in the United States exhibit a certain indifference to the rest of the world. What other country would have the audacity to call its domestic sporting championships the World Series? People in the United States travel abroad far less often than people from other countries. Only about 30 percent of US residents have a passport, compared with around 60 percent of Canadians and 75 percent of people in the United Kingdom (Avon, 2011). This may be a reflection in part of the lack of vacation time enjoyed by the working population outlined in Chapter 4, but it also demonstrates a lack of curiosity about what other nations have to offer. People in the United States might think that they have little to gain from the rest of the world, but given the inferior health conditions in the United States presented in the book, perhaps it is time to look elsewhere to see what lessons can be learned.

We have traced much of what ails people in the United States to the conditions in which people live and work. These problems are exacerbated by the expensive, inefficient US healthcare system dominated by the MIC. The cure for these illnesses may not be easy to achieve. In fact, it may be politically extremely difficult, involving a profound restructuring of power relationships between classes in the United States. Yet conceptually, the solutions are fairly straightforward. Many are successfully in place in other countries. This chapter puts forward three ambitious yet realistic changes to US political economy and healthcare that would drastically improve people's health. The policies are ambitious because they would mark a profound restructuring of the conditions in which people live and work and in their system of healthcare. They are also realistic, having been enacted in other nations. These already existing alternatives are more effective, efficient and egalitarian than the policies currently in place in the United States.

SAFETY FIRST: THE REACH PROGRAM

Both people and the environment are greatly harmed by the side-effects of for-profit modern production processes. This damage is the inevitable result of profit-maximizing firms not being forced to pay the true social costs of their production methods. This is not restricted to the health impacts of pollution problems that economists call externalities, but also includes the unintended results of consuming products with negative side-effects, from prescription drugs to processed foods. The problems associated with some substances, like lead and benzene (and Coca-Cola) are by now well established. Yet the long-term impact of others is not well understood. This is especially true given the complex interactions

Happy birthday?

Coke turned 125 years old in 2011 amid great fanfare and corporate plans to further expand the Coke brand around the globe—although just what isolated corner of the world has yet to learn of its syrupy goodness is a bit of a mystery. Far from celebrating Coke's longevity, Mike Jacobson of the Huffington Post was far from impressed. Coke's list of problematic ingredients starts with high-fructose corn-syrup and continues to: industrial caramel coloring—produced with ammonia and sulfites contaminated with two carcinogens, phosphoric acid that erodes tooth enamel, caffeine, and its cans are lined with the controversial, endocrine-disrupting chemical bisphenol-A. "It's as if this drink were specifically engineered to promote health problems."

According to Jacobson, "Today, 'liquid candy'—non-diet carbonated soft drinks—is the single largest source of American calories, providing about 7 percent of calories. According to our most recent Liquid Candy report, the average 13- to 18-year-old boy drinks about two 12-ounce cans of soda per day; girls of the same age drink the equivalent of one-and-a-third cans per day."

Source: Jacobson (2011).

between different chemicals, and different combinations of those chemicals, and the human body. The difficulty of linking substance *x* to problem *y* in a sufficiently conclusive manner has given rise to two alternative approaches to the problem.

In the United States, substances (except food and drugs) are assumed to be safe unless it can be conclusively proven that they are harmful to humans. This is often made more challenging by business manipulation of the scientific process in defense of their product. Part of this manipulation of science has been lobbying government to reduce its testing and oversight role, as highlighted in a letter from the Union of Concerned Scientists to the United States Department of Agriculture (USDA).

Selections from a letter to USDA Secretary Schafer on NASS, May 20, 2008

Mr. Ed Schafer, Secretary
U.S. Department of Agriculture
1400 Independence Ave., S.W.
Washington, DC 20250

Dear Secretary Schafer:
On behalf of the undersigned organizations and individuals, we are writing to urge you to restore the capacity of the USDA's National Agricultural Statistics Service (NASS) to provide regular and reliable information on agricultural chemical use in the U.S.

NASS has regularly collected and published agricultural chemical use data since at least 1991, but has dramatically scaled back its program in recent years. Now, NASS has taken the most drastic step—announcing that it will not collect agricultural chemical use data on any crops during the 2008 growing season.

NASS's Agricultural Chemical Usage reports are the only reliable, publicly available source of data on pesticide and fertilizer use outside of California. Elimination of this program will severely hamper the efforts of the USDA, the Environmental Protection Agency (EPA), land grant scientists, and state officials to perform pesticide risk assessments and make informed policy decisions on pesticide use.

Agricultural chemical usage data generated by private firms such as Doane or Crop Data Management Systems are both extremely expensive and unreliable, and thus are no substitute for NASS's program. For instance, Doane data cost upwards of $500,000 per year, well beyond the financial resources of our organizations. Even at these prices, the companies severely limit subsequent use and reporting of results derived from analytical work using their data. State governments also find these data too expensive. The EPA, too, has sometimes struggled to find funding to acquire these proprietary data.

NASS's objective and reliable data are critical to sound policy decisions on pesticide use. They are also the only publicly available resource to counter misinformation about pesticide usage and trends in American agriculture.

The undersigned organizations urge you to make every effort to restore NASS's capacity to provide regular and frequent reports on the use of agricultural chemicals in U.S. agriculture. Specifically, we request that NASS reinstate its program of the 1990s, which involved surveys of chemical use annually on major field crops (corn, soybeans, and cotton); periodically on other field crops; and biennially on fruit and vegetable crops.
We look forward to hearing from you.

Among the over 40 organizations to sign the document were the Consumers Union, Greenpeace, the Sierra Club, and the Union of Concerned Scientists.

Source: www.ucsusa.org/food_and_agriculture/science_and_impacts/ science/letter-to-usda-secretary.html (accessed October 11, 2012).

The alternative to the risk assessment principle used in the United States is the precautionary principle, which turns the US presumption of "innocent until proven guilty" on its head by requiring that manufacturers prove that a substance is safe. The logic behind this approach is that uncertainty about the safety of a specific product is not a justification for leaving it on the market. As one review of the literature on cancer concluded, "we will never be able to study and draw conclusions about the potential interactions of exposure to every possible combination of the nearly 100,000 synthetic chemicals in use today … the number of cancer cases that might be caused by environmental carcinogens is likely quite large due to the ubiquity of carcinogens. Thus, the need to limit exposures to environmental and occupational carcinogens is urgent" (Clapp et al., 2005: 27).

The precautionary principle is guiding new European Union legislation on chemicals under the Registration, Evaluation and Authorisation of Chemicals (REACH) program, enacted in 2007. It contains several improvements over the way chemicals are treated in the United States. All substances sold in Europe have to be registered, which requires increasingly stringent toxicity testing with the quantity of the product sold. It is, so far, the "largest effort in history to collect comprehensive toxicity data for chemicals" (Sachs, 2009: 1,835). Without the toxicity data, the product is not allowed to be sold in Europe. The drawback of this scheme, of course, is that the data are provided by industry, but it does improve on the US system that only collects data on those few substances that the underfunded government can manage to test. For those chemicals that cause cancer, birth defects, or genetic mutations, or are persistent or bioaccumulative in the environment, the burden of proof is also shifted to firms. These chemicals will be given a "sunset date" beyond which they cannot be sold in Europe unless they receive government authorization. The European Union estimates that some 1,400 chemicals (about 5 percent of the total) will require this authorization. The final noteworthy difference between REACH and the US regulatory approach is the incentives for substitution. As part of the authorization process, firms must evaluate the suitability of any substitutes and prepare a timetable for implementation of the replacement if feasible (Sachs, 2009: 1,839–43).

REACH is far from perfect. When it was first proposed in the late 1990s, it was considerably stronger. However, the proposed legislation came under forceful attack from the European chemical industry association (CEFIC). According to its president, Eggert Voscherau, REACH would "de-industrialize Europe" and cause "job losses that are put at hundreds of thousands to up to two million" (Osborne, 2003). The European Union was also pressured by the American Chemistry Council and the US State Department, which claimed that REACH would be "unworkable in its implementation, [would] disrupt global trade, and adversely impact innovation" (Chernomas and Hudson, 2007: 101).

The chemical industry has made much of how much REACH would cost to implement. Industry studies estimated these costs at $19 billion (13 billion euros) over eleven years, but other organizations have put forward much lower estimates. The European Union placed the eleven-year costs at $3.3 billion (2.3 billion euros). A study by the Global Development and Environment Institute at

Tufts University estimated $5 billion (3.5 billion euros). However, these costs need to be put in perspective. Even an upper range cost of $1.4 billion per year, almost that provided by the industry study, would represent only 0.2 percent of yearly industry revenues of the European chemical industry (Sachs, 2009: 1,843). Further, in implementing REACH, the European Union anticipates that many of the costs would be offset over time by profits generated from safer alternatives. More importantly, the European Union estimates that it would save $60 billion in chemical-related health costs alone over the next three decades (Chernomas and Hudson, 2007: 102).

The final REACH legislation was the result of a protracted and often acrimonious negotiation between the European Union and industry, but unlike recent US legislation, where it is business that has dominated the political process, REACH is a substantial progressive advance on previous regulation. It seems that, at least in Europe, a new cost–benefit analysis is being undertaken where a more complete social and economic analysis of toxic substances is being incorporated into a new regulatory regime. Catching the source of chronic diseases upstream before it reaches our bodies is an effective and efficient alternative to the current, unenviable US system.

Kids and chemicals

The world is a dangerous place for children. They frequently take what, to adults, would be considered unwise risks with their health in a wide variety of voluntary behaviors, from jumping off roofs to licking unsavory substances. However, many of the most dangerous conditions facing children are hidden and unseen. A recent study concluded that "the costs of lead poisoning, prenatal methylmercury exposure, childhood cancer, asthma, intellectual disability, autism, and attention deficit hyperactivity disorder were $76.6 billion in 2008." With costs of chemical exposure of that magnitude, it is difficult to believe that a program following the REACH principles would not pass a cost–benefit test in the United States. As the authors of the study concluded, "to prevent further increases in these costs, efforts are needed to institute premarket testing of new chemicals; conduct toxicity testing on chemicals already in use; reduce lead-based paint hazards; and curb mercury emissions from coal-fired power plants" (Trasande and Liu, 2011).

EQUALITY, ECONOMIC GROWTH, AND HEALTH

In Chapter 4, we pointed out that one of the important drivers of poor US health is inequality. This is true at the broad societal level, in which the United States ranks as the most unequal nation in the developed world. It is also true at the workplace level, where insecurity, hazardous working conditions and lack of control at the lower ends of the job ladder contribute to poor health. It is well established that those at the lower ends of the societal pecking order have worse health results. This can produce some eye-opening statistics. For example, if the black population in the United States had the same mortality rate as whites, 886,202 deaths would have been avoided between 1991 and 2000 (WHO, 2008a).

The obvious solution to this problem is to reduce inequality. The United States does not have glaring income inequality because of some inevitable national quirk or irreversible economic coincidence. Its inequality is because of deliberate policy actions. Other nations, with different economic policies and political priorities, have achieved much lower inequality.

Although the US government has very occasionally acknowledged the link between inequality and health, it has taken little recent, systematic action to reduce inequality. In 2011, the Department of Health and Human Services issued a report calling for a reduction in health disparities by changing the conditions "where people live, labor, learn, play and pray" (Neergaard, 2010). Yet the House passed a bill later in 2011 that would repeal part of the ACA that promised $15 billion in public health measures, including programs to reduce obesity and improve nutrition—although in a uniquely US twist, President Obama vetoed the repeal (American Press, 2011). The Health Leads program is an example of the US dysfunctional response to the negative health outcomes caused by inequality. It uses volunteers to staff resource desks at 23 hospitals and health centers across the United States to fill physicians' "prescriptions" for food assistance or better shelter. These volunteers use their "problem-solving skills" to identify where the patients might be able to access these much-needed resources (Bornstein, 2011). On one hand this kind of program correctly identifies societal disparities as a crucial determinant of overall health. On the other, most countries would not rely on a staff of college volunteers pointing destitute patients towards insufficient public resources as a solution to health inequality.

There are a number of other ways to deal with inequality. The most obvious is through the tax and transfer system. All developed world countries have a tax system that, at least conceptually, is progressive, which means that it taxes people an increasing proportion of their incomes as their income increases. Tax revenue can then be transferred to lower-income individuals through a variety of programs like income and food supports for the poor. Table 6.1 shows the Gini coefficient for three countries before and after the government intervenes with taxes and transfers. What is immediately apparent is that in all of the countries, incomes are much more equal after taxes and transfers than they were before. It is also true that in all of the countries income inequality has worsened in the last two decades, so the factors that have led to increasing income inequality in the United States were present in other countries as well. However, Table 6.1 shows that the United States does less to redistribute income than other countries. While the US Gini coefficient (before tax and transfer) is not much different from other nations, after taxes and transfers it is much more unequal. Wealth in all nations is even more unequally distributed than income. Table 6.2 shows that wealth is very highly concentrated, but that it is much more concentrated in the United States than it is in Sweden, especially for financial assets.

Sweden has used its tax and transfer system to ensure that far fewer people live below the poverty line than in the United States. In fact, the percentage of the population living in poverty is roughly three times as high in the United States as it is in Sweden (see Table 6.3). The high US poverty rate, and the miserly government transfers that help create it, exist despite the successful example of the Social Security program in the United States. Social Security payments to the elderly were enacted in 1935, and there were substantial increases in benefits in the period following the Second World War. Between 1967 and 2000, the poverty rate (the percentage of the

Table 6.1 Gini coefficients before and after taxes and transfers: total population

Country	Mid-1980s		Mid-2000s	
	Before	**After**	**Before**	**After**
Canada	0.4	0.29	0.44	0.32
Sweden	0.4	0.2	0.43	0.23
United States	0.44	0.34	0.49	0.38

Source: OECD.statextracts Income Distribution Inequality, accessed August 3, 2011.

Table 6.2 Gini coefficients of household net worth, early 2000s

Country	Net worth	Financial assets
Canada	0.67	0.87
Sweden	0.62	0.78
United States	0.77	0.89

Source: Jantti, Siermiknska and Smeeding (2008: 17).

population living below the poverty line) for elderly households fell from 28 to 12 percent. A 2004 study published by the National Bureau of Economic Research concluded that this entire dramatic reduction could be explained by increased social security payments (Engelhardt and Gruber, 2004: 20).

Unemployment insurance in Sweden covers a higher percentage of the unemployed at a higher percentage of their previous wage than is the case in the United States. In the United States, unemployment insurance is passive, in that it provides few supports to those that are unemployed, and provides limited levels of financial assistance for fairly brief periods. In the US state-led system, most benefits run out after 26 weeks (although extended benefits are available in states with high unemployment rates). In order to be eligible workers must be laid off through no fault of their own and have earned sufficient wages in the "base period" (usually the first four of the last five calendar quarters) to qualify. The payment while unemployed is usually 50 percent of the worker's employed wage. The average weekly benefit in 1995 was $187. By contrast, as of 2007, Swedish unemployment insurance paid 80 percent of the

Table 6.3 Poverty rates before and after taxes and transfers: total population

	Mid-1980s		Mid-2000s	
	Before	**After**	**Before**	**After**
Canada	23%	12%	25%	12%
Sweden	26%	3%	27%	5%
United States	26%	18%	26%	17%

Note: the poverty rate is defined as 50 percent of the current median income.

Source: OECD.statextracts Income distribution—poverty.

working wage for the first 200 days, 70 percent for the next 100 days, and 65 percent after that. Sweden also has much more active labor market programs, such as retraining and job finding aids (Olsen, 2011: 122). This kind of transfer should improve health directly through increasing the income of the unemployed, but also through reducing the stress and insecurity associated with job loss that is a fundamental feature of the US labor market.

A second method of reducing inequality is through labor market policy that gives more power to lower-wage workers. Examples of these kinds of policies are minimum wages, favorable rules for collective bargaining, full employment, and generous benefits for the unemployed. All of these policies make it possible for workers to negotiate higher wages by improving their bargaining position with their employers. Increased unionization permits workers to band together and bargain as a group, rather than individually, and institutionalizes the threat of a strike to back up worker demands. Reduced duration of unemployment, through full employment policies, and increased non-labor income, through employment insurance benefits, increases worker bargaining power by decreasing the negative consequences of being without a job.

To provide one example of a policy that would improve the workers' bargaining position, Sweden has a very different union history from the United States. Chapter 4 traced the decline in unionization rates in the United States to changes in government policy and corporate movement to regions with legislation more hostile to unions. Although union solidarity in Sweden has come under pressure by many of the same forces that have caused its decline in the United States, there are still remarkable differences between the two countries. Table 6.4 shows that in 2007, 71 percent of the Swedish labor force belonged to unions compared with only 12 percent in the United States. Further, this understates the number of workers that were covered by collective agreements in Sweden.

Table 6.4 Unionization rates

	Sweden	United States
1980	78%	22%
1990	80%	15%
2007	71%	12%

Source: Olsen (2011: 186).

The coverage rate in 2003 in the United States was 12 percent, but was 93 percent in Sweden, where centralized union bargaining by powerful unions set the working conditions for many non-unionized workers (Olsen, 2011: 187).

Sweden's more unionized workforce not only creates a more egalitarian society in terms of overall income distribution, and as we suggested in Chapter 4, more universal government policies, like public healthcare, that are likely to improve health. It also alleviates some of the powerlessness and lack of control that were highlighted in Chapter 4 as modern contributors to poor health. Workers in unions have greater democratic input into their work lives through

Social spending and health

As we highlighted at the very beginning of the book, the United States spends more money than other nations on healthcare and yet ranks very poorly in terms of health outcomes. In a comparative study of 30 industrialized countries, Elizabeth Bradley and Lauren Taylor argue that if the definition of health spending is broadened to include "social services, like rent subsidies, employment-training programs, unemployment benefits, old-age pensions, family support and other services that can extend and improve life," other countries spend more that the United States. In 2005 the United States devoted 29 percent of GDP to health and social services combined, while countries "like Sweden, France, the Netherlands, Belgium and Denmark dedicated 33 percent to 38 percent of their G.D.P. to the combination." In addition, the United States is one of only three countries to spend the majority of its health and social services budget on healthcare rather than social services. Bradley and Taylor found that countries with low social spending relative to healthcare had lower life expectancy and higher infant mortality than peer countries that reversed these priorities. They conclude:

It is Americans' prerogative to continually vote down the encroachment of government programs on our free-market ideology, but recognizing the health effects of our disdain for comprehensive safety nets may well be the key to unraveling the "spend more, get less" paradox. Before we spend even more money, we should consider allocating it differently.

Source: Bradley and Taylor (2011).

the collective bargaining process. Samuel Bowles (1991) argued that unions could improve people's capacity for the complicated and collective decision-making processes required to fully participate in a democracy (see also Zweig, 2000: 166–7). Workers in unions also have greater security and freedom from arbitrary decisions by their superiors in the workplace. The discussion in Chapter 4 would suggest that the United States might improve its health outcomes by reversing its de-unionization trend.

The final, perhaps least obvious, method of redistributing income is through universal provision of public services. Sweden has much more generous policies than does the United States. In stark contrast to the United States, social welfare programs are universal, rather than means tested. To provide just one example, state-regulated or financed family policies in Sweden are far more all-encompassing. All parents who are either working or in school get access to childcare for their children under 7 years old. They get 16 months of parental leave at 80 percent of their working income. Fathers get ten days of leave after the birth of a child. They also get a further 60 sickness days per child under the age of 12 to allow them to stay home and care for their children. The entire working population receives five weeks of mandatory vacation. On top of this, post-secondary education is free (Olsen, 2011: 122). It is also clear that the kinds of universal family-friendly policies could go some way to alleviating the stress and insecurity that go hand in hand with raising a child on a modest income in the United States.

Further, the fact that universality is a standard feature of Swedish social welfare, and seen as a fundamental right of citizenship, contributes to a shared sense of inclusion in society, which inequality scholars have found improves health outcomes. Table 6.5 highlights the differences between the United States and Sweden (along with Canada, which has universal public healthcare but only a slightly more generous version of US social welfare policy).

In Chapter 4 we presented evidence demonstrating that more equal countries are healthier. There is also evidence that a more powerful labor movement, which in many European countries was the driving force behind the policies that led to a more equal society, is also associated with better health outcomes. A study testing the correlation between various measures of working-class power (union density, years of social democratic government, percentage of "left" votes) and health outcomes (mortality and birth survival) across wealthy nations found a strong positive relationship (Muntaner et al., 2004: 424).

Table 6.5 Ranking on selected social determinants of health among developed
nations

Measure	United States	Canada	Sweden
Percentage in child poverty	22 of 23	17	1
Income inequality	18 of 21	13	3
Percentage in low-paying employment	24 of 24	20	1
Public social spending	28 of 29	23	1
Public share of health spending	20 of 26	23	1
Life expectancy	20 of 26	5	4
Infant mortality	24 of 30	16	1
Child injury mortality	23 of 26	18	1

Source: Raphael (2003).

One of the common objections to increasing equality is that by taxing the rich and giving to the poor, the economy will suffer. Yet there are reasons to believe that a more equal society, with more universal public services can actually increase a nation's competitiveness. The World Economic Forum (WEF) is a Geneva-based foundation whose annual meeting of chief executives and political leaders, held in Davos, Switzerland is a gathering of the truly rich and powerful. The WEF is a think tank funded by 1,000 corporations. Member companies must have annual revenues of more than $1 billion. Every year the WEF produces its *Global Competitiveness Report*, which ranks the competitiveness of the world's economies.

The top ten countries of the WEF Growth Competitiveness Index rankings for 2011 in rank order were Switzerland, Sweden, Singapore, the United States, Germany, Japan, Finland, Netherlands, Denmark, and Canada (Schwab, 2010: 15). What is most interesting about this list is how many of these countries have strong rules that contribute to equality. This is not a one-year anomaly; European countries with generous redistributive policies have fared well in the WEF competitiveness rankings year after year. In 2005 the report lauded these nations for the quality of their public institutions, budget surpluses, low levels of corruption, and high degree of technological innovation. Although these states had high taxes and a strict regulatory framework, they were characterized as having "excellent macroeconomic management overall," according to Augusto Lopez-Carlos, chief economist at the WEF:

> Integrity and efficiency in the use of public resources means there is money for investing in education, in public health, in state-of-the-art infrastructure, all of which contributes to boost productivity. Highly trained labor forces, in turn, adopt new technologies with enthusiasm or, as happens often in the Nordics, are themselves in the forefront of technological innovations. In many ways the Nordics have entered virtuous circles where various factors reinforce each other to make them among the most competitive economies in the world, with world class institutions and some of the highest levels of per capita income in the world.
>
> (Lopez-Carlos, 2005)

Early economic studies suggested that equality-increasing redistribution slowed economic growth, which was harmful even for the poorer recipients of the transfers in the long run (see for example Arrow, 1979; Okun, 1975). However, more recent research has dismissed this connection. It is true that over the last two decades, the United States has grown more than Sweden, yet over the past decade the Nordic nations have had stronger economic growth than the more unequal Anglo countries (the United States, Canada, the United Kingdom) (Olsen, 2011: 95). A 2002 OECD report concluded that there is no evidence that equality affects GDP "one way or another" (Arjona, Ladaique, and Pearson, 2002: 28).

In some ways greater equality would be easy to achieve. Greater redistribution through the tax and transfer system, an alteration of labor market policy and improved universal programs would go a considerable way to easing many of the health problems caused by inequality and insecurity. The Nordic countries, like Sweden, demonstrate that it is possible to implement these kinds of policies and still maintain a competitive economy (Olsen, 2011: 96). Further, the WHO Commission on Social Determinants of Health argued that "Nordic countries, for example, have followed policies that encouraged equality of benefits and services, full employment, gender equity and low levels of social exclusion. This, said the Commission, is an outstanding example of what needs to be done everywhere." According to Sir Michael Marmot, the Commission

The National Nurses United Campaign to Heal America

The United States is hurting. Large banks and other Wall Street firms raided our economy, leaving millions of Americans to suffer. Around the world, poverty, hunger and HIV/AIDS threaten global health.

RNs' duty as patient advocates compels a response: the Nurses Campaign to Heal America.

No matter how the U.S. Supreme Court rules, our health care system will remain broken. We fight for an improved Medicare-for-All system where everyone—rich or poor, young or old—has access to the same standard of safe medical care. Patients' needs must trump insurance coverage.

It's a simple idea: add a tiny sales tax on Wall Street trades that will generate $350 billion a year. The tax—50 cents on every $100 of trades—can help fund social services and rebuild our communities.

Taxpayers bailed out Wall Street. It's time they paid us back.

Working class people are suffering in this economic crisis while the rich grow wealthier and politicians do nothing. The Robin Hood tax can help jump-start a new Economy for the 99% that improves jobs, healthcare, education, retirement and the environment.

(National Nurses United, n.d.)

chair, health policy needs to focus on "creating the conditions for people to be empowered, to have freedom to lead flourishing lives" (WHO, 2008a).

UNIVERSAL, SINGLE-PAYER, PUBLIC HEALTH INSURANCE IN CANADA

The US healthcare system relies more on private, for-profit delivery of both insurance and services than other developed countries. The disappointing results of this approach were highlighted in Chapter 5. It has historically not guaranteed access to millions of its citizens who are uninsured, and even under the ACA, people will still be deterred from seeking medical care because of the payments associated with private insurance. It is also a very expensive system. Similar health results have been achieved with much lower costs in systems that rely less on for-profit delivery within the United States and in other nations. There are a wide variety of alternative mixtures of public and private, profit and non-profit ownership models in different countries, but one of the starkest contrasts with the US system comes from its neighbor, Canada.

Canadian health insurance (Medicare) is paid for out of tax revenue and administered by the government of each province. Comprehensive coverage—which essentially means all necessary hospital and physicians' costs—is provided to all citizens, who also have the option of purchasing supplemental private insurance. Unlike the US system, there is no cost sharing at the point of service. Canadians purchase supplementary private insurance because, depending on the specific provisions in each province, Medicare does not cover some drug costs, dental care, home care, and vision care.

Single-payer national health insurance for the United States as envisioned by the Physicians for a National Health Program

Single-payer national health insurance is a system in which a single public or quasi-public agency organizes health financing, but delivery of care remains largely private.

Currently, the U.S. health care system is outrageously expensive, yet inadequate.

Under a single-payer system, all Americans would be covered for all medically necessary services, including: doctor, hospital, preventive, long-term care, mental health, reproductive health care, dental, vision, prescription drug and medical supply costs. Patients would retain free choice of doctor and hospital, and doctors would regain autonomy over patient care.

Physicians would be paid fee-for-service according to a negotiated formulary or receive salary from a hospital or nonprofit HMO/group practice. Hospitals would receive a global budget for operating expenses. Health facilities and expensive equipment purchases would be managed by regional health planning boards.

A single-payer system would be financed by eliminating private insurers and recapturing their administrative waste. Modest new taxes would replace premiums and out-of-pocket payments currently paid by individuals and business. Costs would be controlled through negotiated fees, global budgeting and bulk purchasing.

(PHNP, n.d.)

Service delivery in Canada is also heavily influenced by provincial governments. The ministers of health control hospital costs by approving and funding global operating budgets for individual hospitals. New facilities and equipment must also be approved and largely funded centrally from the same authority. This institutional arrangement has enabled Canada to contain the escalation of hospital costs relative to the United States. Physicians' fees are determined by means of bilateral monopoly negotiations between provincial medical associations and the ministries of health. Canadian physicians are not permitted to charge patients for anything extra: in other words the government fees represent payment in full. With the price fixed, provincial governments have set up committees to review the patterns of practice so as to identify physicians, and possibly regulate the activities of those who have practices significantly larger than the norm. In addition, some provinces have negotiated aggregate limits on physician billings.

In demonstrating the shortcomings of the current US health system, we provided some evidence on its inefficiency and lack of access in Chapter 5. The private, for-profit portion of the US system fares poorly in comparison with both the public portion of the US system and the Canadian system described above. A single-payer public health system is generally viewed to be superior to a multi-payer private system in terms of both efficiency and equity. Single-payer public systems can raise financing, administer claims, and spread risks over the population more efficiently than a multi-payer private system (Evans, 2000). A tax-financed single-payer system "combines in one authority both the incentive and capacity to contain costs, to a greater degree that is possible in any of the other financing mechanism" (Evans, 2002: 17). Moreover, there are no "marketing expenses, no cost of estimating risk status in order to set differential premiums or decide whom to cover, and no allocations for shareholder profits" (Evans et al., 1989: 573). A comparative analysis of the healthcare costs in the OECD countries found that total healthcare expenditures are lower on average in systems predominantly funded through general taxation (OECD, 2002).

We have already seen that overall healthcare costs are lower in countries with universal public insurance. Part of the reason for this decreased overall cost is reduced spending on healthcare administration. A study comparing the administrative costs (the amount above that paid out for medical care) of the US and Canadian healthcare systems found that 5.9 percent of total healthcare costs in the United States went to insurance administration compared with 1.9 percent in Canada. Further, within the United States, the overhead of private insurance was 11.7 percent compared with 3.6 percent for Medicare and 6.8 percent for Medicaid (Woolhandler, Campbell, and Himmelstein, 2003; see also Himmelstein and Woolhandler, 2008). Other studies have found that administrative costs account for nearly half of the difference between the share of resources allocated to the health sector in the two countries (Himmelstein and Woolhandler, 1986; Fuchs and Hahn, 1990; Himmelstein, Lewontin, and Woolhandler, 1996).

There are additional costs to having private insurance as well. Businesses have to dedicate time and effort to administering healthcare plans. US businesses spent $57 per capita on healthcare consultants and the administrative costs of running their healthcare plans. Canadian firms spent a much more modest $8 per capita on administering health benefits and supplemental private insurance (Woolhandler et al., 2003). Not only is a shift in the financing mix towards a multi-payer private system and away from a tax-financed systems associated with higher costs, it also means a more regressive distribution of payment burden. To the extent that insurance premiums are related to the risk of illness and that the users of care are required to make some financial contributions in the form of deductibles and co-insurance, such a shift in the financing mix involves some transfer of funds from the unhealthy and poor to the healthy and wealthy (Evans, 2000).

In 1991, the CBO released two reports on the feasibility of implementing a single-payer public health insurance system. One compared the saving from two alternative reforms to US healthcare. Both reforms would apply Medicare's rates for all medical services and provide universal insurance. The first would do so while retaining the US system of multiple public and private insurance providers. The second would do so under a single-payer system. Under either reform, "all US residents might be covered by health insurance for roughly the current level of spending or even somewhat less, because of savings in administrative costs and lower payment rates for services used by the privately insured" (CBO, 1991a: 39). Further, the CBO found that, of the two reforms, a single-payer plan would create greater savings. The major drawback of the single-payer system was the possibility that "high-income people would probably pay more for coverage that might be less comprehensive than their current plans," which lays bare the distributional consequences of the health insurance debate (CBO, 1991a: 37).

The second study explicitly drew lessons for the United States from Canada's experience with health insurance. It concluded that "If the US were to shift to a system of universal coverage and a single payer, as in Canada, the savings in administrative costs would be more than enough to offset the expense of universal coverage" (CBO, 1991b: 6). This included not only expanding coverage to those without insurance but also eliminating co-payments and deductibles.

It is not only the CBO that has found the Canadian system more cost-effective. In a *New York Times* op-ed, Bruce Bartlett found that although the United States had one of the lowest tax to GDP ratios (26.1, compared with Canada's 32.3) in the developed world, when healthcare spending is added to get a tax plus healthcare spending-to-GDP ratio, the United States (34.7) is virtually identical to Canada (35.4) (Bartlett, 2011). It is crucial to remember that this similar number funds a more generous social welfare regime in Canada. A study on heart surgery found that it was 83 percent more expensive in the United States than in Canada. Despite the higher US costs, there was no difference in hospital mortality and Canadians remained in the hospital for 17 percent longer (Eisenberg et al., 2005). According to the Medicare Payment Advisory Board, the $24,000 paid to hospitals for each procedure provides about $9,600 in marginal profit on each patient (Barry and Hallam, 2005). More generally, prices in US healthcare are higher than in other countries. This is because in other countries much of the purchasing is either centralized in the hands of the state (as in Canada) or regulated (Germany) (Marmor et al., 2009: 487). A review of studies comparing health outcomes in the two countries found that healthcare spending per patient was 89 percent higher in the United States than in Canada because of Canada's single-payer system for physician and hospital care (Guyatt et al., 2007).

These increased healthcare costs are not associated with superior results. It is a well-established fact that Canada has better broad, more equal health outcomes. According to the Guyatt et al. (2007) review, Canada "produces health benefits similar, or perhaps superior, to those of the US health system." The United States has a higher rate of prematurity and lower birth weight than Canada. A higher percentage of women receive no prenatal care in the first trimester in the United States (16 percent) than in Canada. Better access to healthcare in Canada explains a great deal of the Canadian superiority in heart disease over the United States. Even more convincingly, all of these Canadian advantages only appeared after the passage of national health insurance in that country. Canada has a lower age-adjusted death rate from all cancers (except colorectal) than the United States. The difference in comparable preventable hospitalization rates between rich and poor neighborhoods is much greater in cities in the United States than in publically insured Canada (Billings, Anderson, and Newman, 1996). Finally, health inequalities between the top 10 percent and bottom 10 percent of the income earners are greater in the United States than in Canada (Himmelstein and Woolhandler, n.d.).

This is not to say that there are no critics of the Canadian system. Progressive forces push for the Canadian single-payer system to be expanded to cover a broader range of services, including all drugs and home care. From the other side, conservative forces want hospital and physician services privatized. Some private clinics have been permitted in some provinces. Those who would like to see a greater private role in Canada's public system generally point to two problems. The first is the sustainability of the system. As in all industrialized countries Canadian health expenditures have grown over time. According to the Canadian Health Services Research Foundation, Canada spent 9.8 percent of its GDP on healthcare in 2007, up from 7.1 percent in 1971. Yet, in 2007 France and Germany, with their parallel public and private systems, spent 11.1 and 10.7 percent of their GDP on healthcare respectively (Chernomas, 2010). And we have seen that the United States spends considerably more.

The Canadian healthcare system is part public and part private. Organizationally, hospitals and doctors are privately run, but publicly funded, and must be not-for-profit. Since 1971, the first year of the full implementation of the Canadian Medicare system, expenditures on hospitals, administration, and doctors have remained stable at between 4 and 5 percent of GDP. From 1975 to 2005, hospital expenditures under the publicly funded system have dropped from 44.7 percent of the health budget to 29.9 percent, while spending on doctors has dropped from 15.1 percent to 12.8 percent. The publicly financed parts of the system are clearly a source of sustainability. The source of increased healthcare expenditures is the private for-profit sector, largely outside the scope of the public system. For example, drug expenditures have increased from 8.8 percent of the healthcare budget in 1975 to 17.5 percent in 2005 and have tripled their share of GDP over the past two decades (Chernomas, 2010; see also Evans, 2005; Sepehri and Chernomas, 2004).

In 2002, Ford, GM, and Daimler-Chrysler sent a Joint Letter on

Publicly Funded Health Care to the Canadian government urging that its national healthcare system be "preserved and renewed." The letter praised Canadian Medicare for its affordability, its universal access, the fact that it contributed to a healthier and more productive work force, and created labor cost advantages. It further argued for strengthening the public system to cover drugs and home care (General Motors, Ford and Daimler-Chrysler and the Canadian Auto Workers, 2002).

Opponents of Canadian Medicare often speculate that some province is going to spend 50 percent of its expenditure on healthcare at some time in the future. Such a number should always be treated with suspicion. It often reflects the fact in the neoliberal era provinces have made relatively severe cuts to other social programs so that healthcare expenditures look proportionally large even if they have not changed at all. Similarly, taxes have been cut so much that health expenditure has increased relative to tax revenue. Cutting taxes enough will make any public program unsustainable regardless of how much more efficient it is to run than a private program. In the words of internationally renowned health economist from the University of British Columbia, Robert Evans, "Opponents of Medicare claim that public healthcare is 'Fiscally Unsustainable' and that the only viable solution is a shift to more private coverage. Bluntly, this is a lie" (Evans, 2010).

The second most common complaint revolves around waiting times. In some provinces, private clinics have been allowed as a method to alleviate this problem, but two-tier healthcare systems do not work. England and New Zealand have parallel private healthcare systems and longer waiting times in the public system than countries with a single-payer system such as Canada. In Manitoba, researchers found that the wait for cataract surgery was ten weeks for surgeons who worked exclusively in the public sector and 26 weeks for surgeons who worked in both the public and private systems.

Recognition of this tendency has led the Netherlands to separate their private and public hospitals so that the rich who use the private system cannot use the public one. Sweden, Greece, and Italy also prohibit practice in both systems. Other countries use different ways to achieve the same results. France prohibits doctors in private practice from charging more than they would in the public system. Allowing parallel private systems does not increase existing resources (like the number of doctor and nurses) in healthcare. Rather, it shifts them from the public system to the private, lowering the waiting list in one place while raising it in the other, and shifting health resources from the poor to the rich (Canadian Health Services Research Foundation, 2005; for a discussion of publicly funded, not-for-profit, low-cost alternatives for reducing the problem of waiting lists in Canada see Rachlis, 2004).

Bernie Sanders' solution to high prescription drug prices

Drugs are expensive. Prescriptions can sell for hundreds or even thousands of dollars. Yet these same drugs are remarkably cheap to manufacture. Drug prices are high because lengthy government-granted patent protection, designed to act as an incentive for companies to undertake costly research and development, creates artificial monopolies for individual drugs. According to Dean Baker from the Center for Economic and Policy Research, Senator Bernie Sanders has proposed a clever alternative to this costly and inefficient method of fostering innovation by introducing competition back into the drug industry.

He would establish a government "fund that would buy up patents, so that drugs could then be sold at their free market price. Sanders' bill would appropriate 0.55 percent of GDP (about $80 billion a year, with the economy's current size) for buying up patents, which would then be placed in the public domain so that any manufacturer could use them at no cost." The fund would be created by a levy on insurance companies, which would recoup their increased taxes from the savings they would enjoy because of reduced drug prices. The United States spent an estimated $300 billion on prescription drugs in 2011. Under Sanders' program, "prices would fall to roughly one-tenth this amount in the absence of patent monopolies, leading to savings of more than $250 billion."

Eliminating the patent monopoly would also decrease the incentive for drug companies to engage in some of their more dubious marketing practices, like "overstating the benefits of their drugs and concealing potentially harmful side effects," which have created so many of the recent scandals and controversies in the industry.

The Centers for Medicare and Medicaid Research estimate that over the next ten years the United States will spend "almost $10,000 for every man, woman and child in the country" on prescription drugs. "It's long past time that we did some serious thinking to ensure that we are getting good value for this money."

Source: Baker (2011).

The Canadian healthcare system is far from perfect. Yet it is measurably superior to that currently in place in the United States, even with the passage of the ACA. It is more equal, has universal access and delivers similar results at a fraction of the cost. Canada is not a nation associated with particularly progressive economic or social policies. Most analysts place it firmly in the free market Anglo camp along with the United States, and contrast it with the stronger social programs offered in Europe, especially the Nordic nations. However, Canadian support for its healthcare system is so strong that governments fear being associated with anything that can be labeled US-style healthcare. It is a remarkable political failing that the United States cannot follow the lead of its northern neighbor.

CONCLUSION

On one level, creating a healthier society by implementing the recommendations in this final chapter (or similar alternatives—this is hardly an exhaustive list of the possibilities) would be fairly simple. First, create a more egalitarian society using a combination of tax and transfers, labor market policy, and expanded universal public services. Second, improve the regulatory capacity of agencies that protect people's health, similar to the REACH policy in Europe. Third, implement a public, tax-funded, universal system of health insurance and reduce for-profit ownership of healthcare services. All three of these policies have been implemented elsewhere. Two of the three (REACH is the exception) are long-standing and have been very successful. Infectious disease was defeated only when the conditions that caused the epidemic, such as low wages and unhealthy environments, were addressed. The same is true of the current epidemic of chronic disease. Enacting the three policies in this chapter is not a cure-all that would end chronic disease, but it would mark a substantial improvement on the current policy environment.

These policies would unquestionably represent a 180-degree turn from the general direction of US policy over the last 30 years. Yet as we have seen in Chapters 4 and 5, continuing down the slippery slope that is current US economic and health policy would result in worsening health and earlier mortality. The food people eat, the environment in which they live, and the conditions of their work would continue to cause chronic disease. The negative health impacts of inequality would continue to torment those at the lower ends of the income spectrum. While no healthcare system could possibly compensate for these problems, the current system in the United States is singularly poorly equipped to do so. The ACA may have improved access but it has done little, if anything, to improve the affordability of healthcare for families, the government or firms.

There are groups in the United States striving to enact policies like the three just listed. The example of environmental groups, the Steelworkers, and the American Lung Association coming together as the National Clean Air Coalition to press for the revised Clean Air Act is only one of many examples of the kinds of coalition that have sprung up to press for greater equality, a cleaner environment and more accessible healthcare. So, there are forces in the United States that are pressing for exactly the kinds of policy that have been enacted in other nations.

Yet on another level, implementing any one of these policies, let alone all three of them, would appear to be highly unlikely given the political and economic realities in the United States. There is little evidence on the horizon that a nation that has failed to pass any meaningful progressive legislation in over 30 years is about to start now. However, it might be worth at least pointing out that the reason this is the case is not the frequently heard, and positively framed, arguments about economic efficiency or the political preferences of people in the United States. Rather, it is because of the current power relationships in the economic and political system, in which business has become by far the most effective player, overwhelming the interests of the majority of the population.

As the WHO stated, tackling the "corrosive effects of inequality of life chances" requires us to address "the inequitable distribution of power, money and resources" (WHO, 2008a).

BIBLIOGRAPHY

Akerloff, G. (1970) "The market for 'lemons': quality uncertainty and the market mechanism," *Quarterly Journal of Economics*, Vol. 84, No. 3.

Allen, R. (1994) "Real incomes in the English speaking world," in G. Grantham and M. MacKinnon (eds.), *Labour Market Evolution*. New York: Routledge.

American Cancer Society (2010) *Cancer Facts and Figures 2010*. Atlanta, Ga.: American Cancer Society.

American Lung Association (ALA) (2011) *Trends in Tobacco Use*, ALA Research and Program Services Epidemiology and Statistics Unit, July.

American Press (2011) "House votes to kill preventive health fund," *CBS News*, April 13. www.cbsnews.com/stories/2011/04/13/ap/politics/main20053774.shtml (accessed August 3, 2011).

Angell, M. (2004) *The Truth About the Drug Companies: How they deceive us and what to do about it*. New York: Random House.

Angell, M. (2010) "Big pharma, bad medicine," *Boston Review*, May/June.

Arjona, R., Ladaique, M., and Pearson, M. (2002) "Social protection and growth," *OECD Economic Studies*, No. 35.

Arrow, K. (1979) "The tradeoff between growth and equity," in H. Greenfield (ed.), *Theory for Economic Efficiency*. Princeton, N.J.: Princeton University Press.

Artazcoz, L., Borrell, C., and Benach, J. (2001) "Gender inequalities in health among workers: the relation with family demands," *Journal of Epidemiology and Community Health*, Vol. 55, No. 9.

Ash, M. et al. (2009) *Justice in the Air: Tracking toxic pollution from America's industries and companies to our states, cities, and neighborhoods*. Amherst, Mass.: University of Massachusetts Political Economy Research Institute.

Avon, N. (2011) "Why more Americans don't travel abroad," CNN Travel, February 4. http://articles.cnn.com/2011-02-04/travel/americans.travel.domestically_1_western-hemisphere-travel-initiative-passports-tourism-industries?_s=PM:TRAVEL (accessed April 10, 2012).

Baird, P. (1994) "The role of genetics in population health," in R. Evans, B. Morris, and T. Marmor (eds.), *Why are Some People Healthy and Others are Not?* New York: Walter de Gruyter.

Baker, D. (2011) "Bernie Sanders tries some clear thinking on prescription drugs," *Huffington Post*, June 1. www.huffingtonpost.com/dean-baker/bernie-sanders-tries-some_b_869778.html (accessed March 2, 2012).

Baker, D. et al. (2001) "Lack of health insurance and decline in overall health in late middle age," *New England Journal of Medicine*, Vol. 345, No.15.

Baldwin, P. (1999) *Contagion and the State in Europe, 1830–1930*. Cambridge: Cambridge University Press.

Baillie-Hamilton, P. (2002) "Chemical toxins: a hypothesis to explain the global obesity epidemic," *Journal of Alternative and Complementary Medicine*, Vol. 8.

Barbeau, E., Leavy-Sperounis, A., and Balbach, E. (2004) "Smoking, social class, and gender: what can public health learn from the tobacco industry about disparities in smoking?" *Tobacco Control*, Vol. 13, No. 2.

Barry, T. and Hallam, K. (2005) "Heart surgery costs 83% more in U.S. than in Canada, study says," *Bloomberg*, July 11. www.bloomberg.com/apps/news?pid=newsarchive&sid=a4J.ER8r4CrM&refer=canada (accessed July 10, 2011).

Bartlett, B. (2011) "What your taxes do (and don't) buy for you," *New York Times*, June 7. http://economix.blogs.nytimes.com/2011/06/07/health-care-costs-and-the-tax-burden/ (accessed August 7, 2011).

Bartley, M., Ferrie, J., and Montgomery, S. (2006) "Health and labour market disadvantage: unemployment, non-employment, and job insecurity," in M. Marmot and R. Wilkinson (eds.), *Social Determinants of Health*. Oxford: Oxford University Press.

Bambra, C. and Eikemo, T. (2008) "Welfare state regimes, unemployment and health: a comparative study of the relationship between unemployment and self-reported health in 23 European countries," *Journal of Epidemiology and Community Health*, Vol. 63, No. 2.

Baxandall, R., Gordon, L., and Reverby, S. (1976) *America's Working Women,* New York: Random House.

Beckfield, J. and Krieger, N. (2009) "Epi + demos + cracy: linking political systems and priorities to the magnitude of health inequities – evidence, gaps, and a research agenda," *Epidemiologic Reviews*, Vol. 31, No. 1.

Berkman, L. and Epstein, A. (2008) "Beyond health care – socioeconomic status and health," *New England Journal of Medicine*, Vol. 358, No. 23.

Bernstein, M. (2009) "Propaganda and prejudice distort the health reform debate," *Health Affairs*, April 22. http://healthaffairs.org/blog/2009/04/22/proganda-and-prejudice-distort-the-health-reform-debate/ (accessed July 15, 2011).

Billings, J., Anderson, G., and Newman, L. (1996) "Recent findings on preventable hospitalizations," *Health Affairs*, Vol. 15, No. 3.

Birn, A-E., Pillay, Y., and Holtz, T. (2009) *Textbook of International Health: Global health in a dynamic world.* New York: Oxford University Press.

Blumberg, L. (2010) "How will the patient protection and affordable care act affect small, medium, and large businesses?" *Timely Analysis of Immediate Health Policy Issues*, Urban Institute.

Blumenfeld, A. (1964) *Heart Attack: Are you a candidate?* New York: Paul S. Erikson.

Blyth, M. (2002) *Great Transformations: Economic ideas and institutional change in the twentieth century.* Cambridge: Cambridge University Press.

Bohme, S., Zorabedian, J., and Egilman, D. (2005) "Maximizing profit and endangering health: corporate strategies to avoid litigation and regulation," *International Journal of Occupational and Environmental Health*, Vol. 11, No. 4.

Bornstein, D. (2011) "Treating the cause, not the illness," *New York Times*, July 28. http://opinionator.blogs.nytimes.com/2011/07/28/treating-the-cause-not-the-illness/ (accessed August 3, 2011).

Bowles, S. (1991) "What markets can – and cannot – do," *Challenge*, Vol. 34, No. 4.

Boyer, G. (2010) "English poor laws," http://eh.net/encyclopedia/article/boyer.poor.laws.england (accessed January 31, 2012).

Braverman, P. et al. (2010) "Socioeconomic disparities in health in the US: what the patterns tell us," *American Journal of Public Health*, Vol. 100, Supp. 1.

Braverman, H. (1974) *Labor and Monopoly Capital: The degradation of work in the twentieth century.* New York: Monthly Review Press.

Brenner, H. (2005) "Commentary: economic growth is the basis of mortality rate decline in the 20th century – experience of the United States 1901–2000," *International Journal of Epidemiology*, Vol. 35.

Brenner, R. (2006) *The Economics of Global Turbulence.* London: Verso.

Brieger, G. (1997) "Sanitary reform in New York City," in J. Leavitt and R. Numbers (eds.), *Sickness and Health in America,* Madison, Wisc.: University of Wisconsin Press.

Brierley, J. (1970) *A Natural History of Man.* New Jersey: Associated University Press.

Brownell, K. (1998) "The pressure to eat," www.cspinet.org/nah/7_98eat.htm (accessed May 23, 2011).

Bryson, B. (2003) *A Short History of Nearly Everything.* Toronto: Anchor Canada.

Buettgens, M., Garrett, B., and Holahan, J. (2010) *America Under the Affordable Health Care Act,.* Washington DC: Urban Institute.

Bureau of Labor Statistics (2012) "The employment situation – December 2011," news release, January 6. www.bls.gov/news.release/pdf/empsit.pdf (accessed January 19, 2012).

Burrow, J. (1977) *Organized Medicine in the Progressive Era.* Baltimore, Md.: Johns Hopkins University Press.

Cairns, E. (1971) *The Biological Imperatives.* New York: Holt, Rinehart & Winston.

Canadian Centre for Policy Alternatives (1998) *CCPA Monitor*, November.

Canadian Health Coalition (2011) *Canadians' Views on Public Healthcare Solutions* http://healthcoalition.ca/wp-content/uploads/2011/11/NANOS-EN.pdf (accessed March 1, 2011).

Canadian Health Services Research Foundation (2005) "Myth: a parallel private system would reduce waiting times in the public system,"

Myth busters, March, www.chsrf.ca/Migrated/PDF/myth17_e.pdf (accessed March 5, 2012).

Carson, R. (1962) *Silent Spring*. New York: Houghton Mifflin.

Casarett, I. and Doull, J. (eds.) (1975) *Toxicology*, New York: Macmillan.

Cassel, E. (1976) *The Healers Art*. Philadelphia, Pa.: J. B. Lippincott.

Centers for Disease Control and Prevention (2010) "Vital signs: current cigarette smoking among adults aged ≥18 Years – United States, 2009." www.cdc.gov/mmwr/preview/mmwrhtml/mm5935a3.htm?s_cid=mm5935a3_w (accessed January 24, 2012).

Center for Responsive Politics (CRP) (2009) "2008 Presidential election contributions by sector," www.opensecrets.org/pres08/sectorall.php?cycle=2008 (accessed July 1, 2010).

CRP (2010) "2010 Overview top industries," www.opensecrets.org/overview/industries.php (accessed July 1, 2011).

CRP (2011) "Lobbying top industries," www.opensecrets.org/lobby/top.php?indexType=i (accessed July 11, 2011).

Chernomas, R. (1999) *The Social and Economic Causes of Disease*. Ottawa, ON: Canadian Centre for Policy Alternatives.

Chernomas, R. (2010) *Profit Is Not the Cure 2010: Is the Canadian economy sustainable without Medicare?* Ottawa, ON: Council of Canadians.

Chernomas, R. and Donner, L. (2004) *The Cancer Epidemic as a Social Event*. Winnipeg, MB: Canadian Centre for Policy Alternatives – Manitoba.

Chernomas, R. and Hudson, I. (2007) *Social Murder and Other Problems with Conservative Economics*. Winnipeg, MB: Arbeiter Ring.

Chren, M., Landefeld, C., and Murray, T. (1989) "Doctors, drug companies and gifts," *Journal of the American Medical Association*, Vol. 262.

Clapp, R., Howe, G., and Jacobs, M. (2007) "Environmental and occupational causes of cancer: a call to act on what we know," *Biomedicine and Pharmacotherapy*, Vol. 61, No. 10.

Clapp, R., Howe, G., and Lefevre, M. (2005) *Environmental and Occupational Causes of Cancer: A review of recent scientific literature*. Lowell, Mass.: Lowell Center for Sustainable Production, University of Massachusetts Lowell.

Clark, J. B. (1899) *The Distribution of Wealth: A theory of wages, interest and profit*. New York: Macmillan.

Cogan, J., Hubbard, R., and Kessler, D. (2006) *Healthy, Wealthy, and Wise: Five steps to a better health care system*. Washington DC: AEI Press.

Cole, P. and Goldman, M. (1975) "Occupation," in J. Fraumeni (ed.), *Persons at High Risk of Cancer*. New York: Academic Press.

Colgrove, J. (2002) "The McKeown thesis: a historical controversy and its enduring influence," *American Journal of Public Health*, Vol. 92, No. 5.

Commins, J. (2010) "Physicians generate $1.5M annually for their hospitals, says survey," *Health Leaders Media*, March 17, www.healthleadersmedia.com/content/FIN-248119/Physicians-Generate-

15M-Annually-for-Their-Hospitals-Says-Survey (accessed February 18, 2012).

Condran, G., Williams, H., and Cheney, R. (1997) "The decline in mortality in Philadelphia from 1870 to 1930: the role of municipal services," in J. Leavitt and R. Numbers (eds.), *Sickness and Health in America*, Madison, Wisc.: University of Wisconsin Press.

Congressional Budget Office (CBO) (1991a) *Universal Health Insurance Coverage Using Medicare's Payment Rates*. Washington DC: US Government Printing Office.

CBO (1991b) *Canadian Health Insurance: Lessons for the United States*, ref. no. HRD-91-90. Washington DC: US Government Printing Office.

CBO (2011a) *Long Term Analysis of a Budget Proposal by Chairman Ryan*. Washington DC: US Government Printing Office.

CBO (2011b) *Letter to Honorable John Boehner, Speaker of the House, January 6, 2011: Review of the H.R. 2, The Repealing the Job-Killing Health Care Law Act*. www.cbo.gov/ftpdocs/120xx/doc12040/01-06-PPACA_Repeal.pdf (accessed September 27, 2011).

Consumer Reports (2000) "Is an HMO for you? Practices of health maintenance organizations," *Consumer Reports*, Vol. 65, No. 7.

Cooper, J. (1980) *The Army and Civil Disorder*. Westport, Conn.: Greenwood Press.

Cornell University ILR School (2011) "The Triangle factory fire 100 years later," www.ilr.cornell.edu/trianglefire/legacy/legislativeReform.html (accessed April 15, 2011).

Cutler, D., Deaton, A., and Lleras-Muney, A. (2006) "The determinants of mortality," *Journal of Economic Perspectives*, Vol. 20, No. 3.

Cutler, D., and Miller, G. (2005) "The role of public health improvements in health advances: the twentieth-century United States," *Demography*, Vol. 42, No. 1.

Davis, D. (2007) *The Secret History of the War on Cancer*. New York: Basic Books.

Davis, D. L. and Rall, D. P. (1981)"Risk assessment for disease prevention," in L. K.Y. Ng and D. L. Davis (eds.), *Strategies for Public Health,* New York, Van Nostrand Reinhold.

Davis, H. (1988) "Reform and the Triangle shirtwaist company fire," *Concord Review*, Vol. 1, No. 1.

DeNavas-Walt, C., Proctor, B., and Smith, J. (2008) *U.S. Census Bureau, Current Population Reports, P60-235, Income, Poverty, and Health Insurance Coverage in the United States: 2007*. Washington DC: US Government Printing Office.

Devereaux, P. et al. (2002) "Comparison of mortality between private for-profit and private not-for-profit hemodialysis centers: a systematic review and meta-analysis," *Journal of the American Medical Association*, Vol. 288, No. 19.

Dorn, S. and Buettgens, M. (2010) *Net Effects of the Affordable Care Act on State Budgets*. Washington DC: Urban Institute.

Dougherty, K. (2007) "Comment: Methanex v. United States: the realignment of NAFTA Chapter 11 with environmental regulation," *Northwest Journal of International Law and Business,* Vol. 27, No. 3.

Dubofsky, M. (1994) *The State and Labor in Modern America.* Chapel Hill, N.C.: University of North Carolina Press.

Dubofsky, M. (1996) *Industrialism and the American Worker: 1865–1920.* Wheeling, Ill.: Harlan Davidson.

Dubois, L. (2006) "Food, nutrition and population health: from scarcity to social inequalities," in J. Heymann et al. (eds.), *Healthier Societies: From Analysis to Action.* Oxford: Oxford University Press.

Dubos, R. (1950) *Louis Pasteur.* Massachusetts: Little, Brown.

Dubos, R. (1959) *Mirage of Health,* ed. Ruth Nanda Anshen. New York: Harper & Brothers.

Dubos, R. (1965) *Man Adapting.* New Haven, Conn.: Yale University Press.

Duffy, J. (1997) "Social role of disease in the late 19th century," in J. Leavitt and R. Numbers (eds.), *Sickness and Health in America.* Madison, Wisc.: University of Wisconsin Press.

Duménil, G. and Lévy, D. (2002) "The profit rate: where and how much did it fall? Did it recover? (USA 1948–2000)," *Review of Radical Political Economy,* Vol. 34, No. 4.

Eggan, D., and Kindy, K. (2009) "Former lawmakers and Congressional staffers hired to lobby on health care," *Washington Post,* July 6.

Egilman, D. and Bohme, S. (2005) "Over a barrel: corporate corruption of science and its effects on workers and the environment," *International Journal of Occupational and Environmental Health,* Vol. 11, No. 4.

EH.net (2001) "Hours of work in US history," http://eh.net/encyclopedia/article/whaples.work.hours.us (accessed 22 October 2012).

Ehrenreich, B. and Ehrenreich, J. (1971) *The American Health Empire: Power, profits and politics.* New York: Vintage.

Eichenwald, K. (1997) "Health care's giant: artful accounting. Hospital chain cheated US on expenses, documents show," *New York Times,* December 18.

Eichenwald, K. (2003) "How one hospital benefited from questionable surgery," *New York Times,* August 12.

Eisenberg, M. J. et al. (2005) "Outcomes and cost of coronary artery bypass graft surgery in the United States and Canada," *Archives of Internal Medicine,* Vol. 165, No. 13.

Engelhardt, G. and Gruber, J. (2004) "Social security and the evolution of elderly poverty," Working Paper 10466. Washington DC: National Bureau of Economic Research.

Engels, F. (1850) *The Conditions of the Working Class in England in 1844.* London: George Allen & Unwin.

Environmental Protection Agency (EPA) (2010) *Our Nation's Air: Status and Trends Through 2008.* Research Triangle Park, N.C.: EPA.

EPA (2011) *The Benefits and Costs of the Clean Air Act from 1990 to 2020.* Washington DC: EPA Office of Air and Radiation.

Environmental Working Group (2003) *Body Burden: The pollution in people.* www.ewg.org/sites/bodyburden1/es.php (accessed March 25, 2011).

Epstein, H. (1998) "Life and death on the social ladder," *New York Review of Books,* Vol. 45, No. 12, July 16.

Epstein, R. (1997) *Mortal Peril: Our inalienable right to health care?* New York: Addison-Wesley.

Epstein, S. (1998) *The Politics of Cancer Revisited.* Fremont Center, N.Y.: East Ridge Press.

Epstein, S. et al. (2002) "Track record of the American Cancer Society: the crisis in U.S. and international cancer policy," *International Journal of Health Services,* Vol. 32, No. 4.

Esping-Anderson, G. (1990) *The Three Worlds of Welfare Capitalism.* Princeton, N.J.: Princeton University Press.

Estes, C., Harrington, C., and Pellow, D. (2000) "Medical-industrial complex," in E. Borgatta and R. Montgomery (eds.), *Encyclopedia of Sociology.* Farmington Hills, Mich.: Gale Group.

Evans, A. (1973) "Pettenkofer revisited: the life and contributions of Max von Pettenkofer (1818–1901)," *Yale Journal of Biology and Medicine,* Vol. 46.

Evans, R. (1984) *Strained Mercy: The economics of Canadian health care.* Toronto: Butterworths.

Evans, R. (1994) "Introduction," in R. Evans, B. Morris, and T. Marmor (eds.), *Why are Some People Healthy and Others are Not?* New York: Walter de Gruyer.

Evans, R. (2000) "Financing health care: taxation and the alternatives," HPRU discussion paper no. 2000:15D. Vancouver, BC: University of British Columbia Center for Health Services and Policy Research (CHSPR).

Evans, R. (2002) "Raising the money: options, consequences, and objectives for financing health care in Canada," discussion paper no. 27, prepared for the Commission on the Future of Health Care in Canada.

Evans, R. (2005) "Political wolves and economic sheep: the sustainability of public health insurance in Canada," Working paper CHSPR 03:16W. Vancouver, BC: CHSPR.

Evans, R. (2010) "Public health care as sustainable as we want it to be," *Toronto Star,* June 1 www.thestar.com/opinion/editorialopinion/article/817249--public-health-care-as-sustainable-as-we-want-it-to-be (accessed March 3, 2012).

Evans, R. et al. (1989) "Controlling health expenditures – the Canadian reality," *New England Journal of Medicine,* Vol. 320, No. 9.

Evans, R. G., Morris, B. L., and Marmor, T. R. (eds.) (1994) *Why are Some People Healthy and Others are Not?* New York: Walter de Gruyter.

Faber, D. and Krieg, E. (2002) "Unequal exposure to ecological hazards: environmental injustices in the Commonwealth of Massachusetts," *Environmental Health Perspectives,* Vol. 110, Supp. 2.

Faguet, G. (2005) *The War on Cancer: An anatomy of failure, a blueprint for the future*. Dordrecht, Netherlands: Springer.

Families USA. (2004) "One in three: non-elderly Americans without health insurance," June 3. www.familiesusa.org/assets/pdfs/82million_uninsured_report6fdc.pdf (accessed July 13, 2011).

Fee, E. (1994) "Public health and the state: the United States," in D. Porter (ed.), *The History of Public Health and the Modern State*. Amsterdam: Editions Rodopi.

Fein, R. (1986) *Medical Care, Medical Costs: The search for a health insurance policy*. Cambridge, Mass.: Harvard University Press.

Feinstein, C. (1998) "Pessimism perpetuated: real wages and the standard of living in Britain during and after the industrial revolution," *Journal of Economic History*, Vol. 58, No. 3.

Feldstein, M. (1973) "The welfare loss of excessive health insurance," *Journal of Political Economy*, Vol. 81, No. 1.

Feldstein, P. (1999) *Health Care Economics*, 5th edn. Albany, N.Y.: Delmar.

Ferrie, J. et al. (1995) "Health effects of anticipation of job change and non-employment: longitudinal data from the Whitehall II study," *British Medical Journal*, Vol. 311, No. 7015.

Finkelstein, A. et al. (2011) "The Oregon health insurance experiment: evidence from the first year," Working Paper No. 17190. Washington DC: National Bureau for Economic Research (NBER).

Fitch, J. (1924) *The Causes of Industrial Unrest*. New York: Harper & Brothers.

Flinn, M. (1965) "Introduction," in E. Chadwick, *Report of the Sanitary Condition of the Labouring Population of Great Britain*. Edinburgh: Edinburgh University Press.

Fogel, R. (1997) "New findings on secular trends in nutrition and mortality: some implications for population theory," in M. R. Rosenzweig and O. Stark (eds.), *Handbook of Population and Family Economics*. New York: Elsevier Science, North Holland.

Fogel, R. (2004) *The Escape from Hunger and Premature Death, 1700–2100*. Cambridge: Cambridge University Press.

Foner, P. (1947) *History of the Labor Movement in the United States Vols 1–4*. New York: International Publishers.

Ford, E. et al. (2007) "Explaining the decrease in U.S. deaths from coronary disease, 1980–2000," *New England Journal of Medicine*, Vol. 356.

Fortune (2009) "Top industries: most profitable," *Fortune 500*, http://money.cnn.com/magazines/fortune/fortune500/2009/performers/industries/profits/ (accessed July 11, 2011).

Frank, J. et al. (2006) "Interactive role of genes and the environment," in J. Heymann et al. (eds.), *Healthier Societies: From analysis to action*. Oxford: Oxford University Press.

Freeman, J. (2009) "A modest proposal: bribe the insurance companies," *Medicine and Social Justice*, August 23. http://medicinesocialjustice.blogspot.com/2009/08/modest-proposal-bribe-insurance.html (accessed August 7, 2011).

Freeman, J. (2012) "The high cost of drugs: treating cancer and cholesterol while building profit," *Medicine and Social Justice*, February 12.
http://medicinesocialjustice.blogspot.com/2012/02/high-cost-of-drugs-
treating-cancer-and.html (accessed February 28, 2012).

Fuchs, V. (1986) *The Health Economy.* Cambridge, Mass.: Harvard
University Press.

Fuchs, V. and Hahn, J. (1990) "How does Canada do it? A comparison of
expenditures for physicians' services in the United States and Canada,"
New England Journal of Medicine, Vol. 323, No. 13.

Gagnon M.-A. and Lexchin, J. (2008) "The cost of pushing pills: a new
estimate of pharmaceutical promotion expenditures in the United
States," *PLoS Medicine*, Vol. 5, No. 1.

Galdston, I. (1954) *The Meaning of Social Medicine.* Boston, Mass.:
Harvard University Press.

Garg, P. et al. (1999) "Effect of the ownership of dialysis facilities on
patients' survival and referral for transplantation," *New England
Journal of Medicine*, Vol. 341, No. 22.

Gawande, A. (2009) "The cost conundrum: what a Texas town can teach
us about health care," *New Yorker*, Vol. 85, No. 16, June 1.

General Motors, Ford and Daimler-Chrysler, and Canadian Auto Workers
(2002) "General Motors, Ford and Daimler-Chrysler and the Canadian
Auto Workers support Canadian medicare: Joint letter on publicly
funded health care," press release, September 12.

Gerth, J. and Stolberg, S. (2000) "Drug makers reap profits on tax-backed
research," *New York Times*, April 23.

Geyman, J. (2003) "Myths as barriers to health care reform in the United
States," *International Journal of Health Services*, Vol. 33, No. 2.

Gimeno, D. et al. (2004) "Psychosocial factors and work related sickness
absence among permanent and non-permanent employees," *Journal of
Epidemiology and Community Health*, Vol. 58, No. 10.

Ginzberg, E. (1977) *The Limits of Health Reform: The search for realism.*
New York: Basic Books.

Gladwell, M. (2005) "The moral hazard myth: the bad idea behind our
failed health care system," *New Yorker*, August 29.

Gonzalez, G. (2001) *Corporate Power and the Environment.* Lanham, Md.:
Rowman & Littlefield.

Gonzalez, G. (2005) *The Politics of Air Pollution.* Albany, N.Y.: State
University of New York Press.

Gordon, D., Bowles, S., and Weisskopf, T. (1994) "Power, profits, and
investment: an institutional explanation of the stagnation of U.S. net
investment after the mid-1960s," New School for Social Research
Working Paper no. 12. Repr. in S. Bowles and T. Weisskopf (eds.),
*Economics and Social Justice: Essays on power, labor and institutional
change.* Cheltenham: Edward Elgar.

Gottlieb, M., Eichenwald, K., and Barbanel, J. (1997) "Biggest hospital
operator attracts federal inquiries," *New York Times*, March 28.

Graham, D. (2004) "Blowing the whistle on the FDA: an interview with Dr. David Graham," *Multinational Monitor*, Vol. 25, No. 12.

Graham, H. (1994) "Gender and class as dimensions of smoking behaviour in Britain: insights from a survey of mothers," *Social Science and Medicine*, Vol. 38, No. 5.

Graham, H. and Der, G. (1998) "Influences on women's smoking status: the contribution of socioeconomic status in adolescence and adulthood," *European Journal of Public Health*, Vol. 9, No. 2.

Greenspan, A. (1997) "Testimony before the committee on the budget," United States Senate, January 21. Washington DC: Federal Reserve Board. www.federalreserve.gov/BOARDDOCS/Testimony/1997/19970121.htm (accessed March 12, 2007).

Griffiths, C., Rooney, C., and Brock, A. (2005) "Leading causes of death in England and Wales: how should we group the causes?" *Health Statistics Quarterly*, Vol. 28.

Grossman, M. (1972) "On the concept of health capital and the demand for health," *Journal of Political Economy*, Vol. 80, No. 2.

Guyatt, G. et al. (2007) "A systematic review of studies comparing health outcomes in Canada and the United States," *Open Medicine*, Vol. 1, No. 1. www.openmedicine.ca/article/view/8/1 (accessed August 7, 2011).

Hacker, D. (2010) "Decennial life tables for the white population of the United States, 1790–1900," *Historical Methods*, Vol. 43, No. 2.

Hacker, J. (2002) *The Divided Welfare State: The battle over public and private social benefits in the United States*. Cambridge: Cambridge University Press.

Heilbroner, R. (1977) *The Economic Transformation of America*. New York: Harcourt Brace Jovanovich.

Heindel, J. (2003) "Endocrine disruptors and the obesity epidemic," *Toxicological Sciences*, Vol. 76, No. 2.

Hemenway, D. et al. (1990) "Physicians' responses to financial incentives – evidence from a for-profit ambulatory care center," *New England Journal of Medicine*, Vol. 322, No. 15.

Hendricks, A., Remler, D., and Prashker, M. (1999) "More or less? Methods to compare VA and non-VA health care costs," *Medical Care*, Vol. 37, No. 4.

Hersh-Cochran, M. (1989) *Compendium of English Language Course Syllabi and Textbooks in Health Economics*. Copenhagen: World Health Organization (WHO) Regional Office for Europe.

Hertzman, C. and Siddiqi, A. (2008) "Tortoises 1 hares 0: how comparative health trends between Canada and the United States support a long term view of health policy," *Healthcare Policy*, Vol. 4, No. 2.

Hileman, B. (2009) "Are contaminants silencing our genes?" *Scientific American*, August 3. www.scientificamerican.com/article. cfm?id=silencing-genes-chemical-contaminants-cancer-diabetes (accessed March 21, 2011).

Hillman, A., Pauly, M., and Kerstein, J. (1989) "How do financial incentives affect physicians' clinical decisions and the financial performance of Health Maintenance Organizations?," *New England Journal of Medicine*, Vol. 321, No. 2.

Hilzenrath, D. (2009) "Health insurance lobby cherry-picks data in fight against public plan," *Washington Post*, July 22.

Himmelstein, D., Lewontin, J., and Woolhandler, S. (1996) "Who administers who cares? Medical administrative and clinical employment in the United States and Canada," *American Journal of Public Health*, Vol. 86, No. 2.

Himmelstein, D. and Woolhandler, S. (1986) "Cost without benefit: administrative waste in U.S. health care," *New England Journal of Medicine*, Vol. 314, No. 7.

Himmelstein, D. and Woolhandler, S. (1995) "Care denied: U.S. residents who are unable to obtain needed medical services," *American Journal of Public Health*, Vol. 85, No. 3.

Himmelstein, D. and Woolhandler, S. (2008) "Privatization in a publicly funded health care system: the US experience," *International Journal of Health Services*, Vol. 38, No. 3.

Himmelstein, D. and Woolhandler, S. (n.d.) "Recent attacks on single payer health reform: ideology masquerading as scholarship," *Single Payer FAQ*. www.pnhp.org/facts/single-payer-faq#response-papers (accessed August 7, 2011).

Hirsch, B. T., Macpherson, D. A., and Vroman, W. G. (2001) "Estimates of union density by state," *Monthly Labor Review*, Vol. 124, No. 7, pp. 51–5 (accompanying data online at www.unionstats.com)

Hobsbawm, E. J. (1964) *Labouring Men*. New York: Basic Books.

Hobsbawm, E. J. (1974) *Industry and Empire*. Harmondsworth: Penguin.

Hobsbawm, E. J. (1975) *The Age of Capital 1848–1875*. London: Weidenfeld & Nicolson.

Hoffman, B. (2001) *The Wages of Sickness: The politics of health insurance in progressive America*. Chapel Hill, N.C.: University of North Carolina Press.

Huff, J. (2007) "Industry influence on occupational and environmental public health," *International Journal of Occupational and Environmental Health*, Vol. 13, No. 1.

Humana (2011) *Annual Report 2010*. Loiusville, Ky.: Humana.

International Agency of Research on Cancer (IARC) (1979) *Chemical and Industrial Processes Associated with Cancer in Humans*, supplement to vols. 1–20, Lyon, IARC.

International Labour Organization (ILO) (2005) *Global Estimates of Fatal Work Related Diseases and Occupational Accidents, World Bank Regions 2005: Established market economies*. www.ilo.org/legacy/english/protection/safework/accidis/globest_2005/index.htm (accessed August 31, 2011).

ILO (2009) *Occupational Injuries: United States, 2009*. http://laborsta.ilo.org/STP/do (accessed April 9, 2009).

Irigaray, P. et al. (2007) "Lifestyle-related factors and environmental agents causing cancer: an overview," *Biomedicine and Pharmacotherapy*, Vol. 61, No. 10.

Isaacson, E. (1993) "Prescription for change," *San Francisco Bay Guardian*, April 14.

Jack, A. (2011) "A sugared pill," *Financial Times*, March 8.

Jackevicius, C. et al. (2012) "Generic atorvastatin and health care costs," *New England Journal of Medicine*, Vol. 366, No. 3.

Jacobson, M. (2011) "Coke turns 125: why I'm not celebrating," *Huffington Post*, May 11.

Jantti, M., Sierminska, E., and Smeeding, T. (2008) "The joint distribution of household income and wealth: evidence from the Luxembourg wealth study," Social, Employment and Migration Working Papers no. 65. Paris: Organisation for Economic Co-operation and Development (OECD).

Jha, A. et al. (2001) "Racial differences in mortality among men hospitalized in the Veterans Affairs Health Care system," *Journal of the American Medical Association*, Vol. 285, No. 3.

Johnson, T. (2010*) Healthcare Costs and U.S. Competitiveness,* Council on Foreign Relations. www.cfr.org/health-science-and-technology/health-care-costs-us-competitiveness/p13325 (accessed June 29, 2011).

Joint Economic Committee, United States Senate (2000) *The Benefits of Medical Research and the Role of the NIH*, 106th Congress 2nd Session. Washington DC, US Senate.

Karasek, R. and Theorell, T. (1990) *Healthy Work, Stress, Productivity and the Reconstruction of Working Life*. New York: Basic Books.

Katz, R. (2012) "Environmental pollution: corporate crime and cancer mortality," *Contemporary Justice Review: Issues in Criminal, Social, and Restorative Justice*, Vol. 15, No.1.

Kawachi, I., Daniels, N., and Robinson, D. (2005) "Health disparities by race and class: why both matter," *Health Affairs*, Vol. 24, No. 2.

Kessler, R., Turner, J., and House, J. (1987) "Intervening processes in the relationship between unemployment and health," *Psychological Medicine*, Vol. 17, No. 4.

Keynes, J. M. (1920) *The Economic Consequences of the Peace*. New York: Harcourt, Brace & Howe.

Keyssar, A. (1986) *Out of Work: The first century of unemployment in Massachusetts*. Cambridge: Cambridge University Press.

Knowles, J. (1977) "The responsibility of the individual," *Daedalus*, Vol. 106, No. 1.

Kolonel, L. and Wilkens, L. (2006) "Migrant studies," in D. Schottenfeld and J. Fraumeni (eds.), *Cancer Epidemiology and Prevention*. Oxford: Oxford University Press)

Kopczuk, W. and Saez, E. (2004) "Top wealth shares in the United States, 1916–2000: evidence from estate tax returns," *National Tax Journal*, Vol. 57, No. 2.

Kraft, M. (2011) *Environmental Policy and Politics*, 5th edn. Boston, Mass.: Longman.

Krause, P. (1992) *The Battle for Homestead 1880–1892: Politics, culture and steel*. Pittsburgh, Pa.: University of Pittsburgh Press.

Krieger, N. (2005) "Embodiment: a conceptual glossary for epidemiology," *Journal of Epidemiology and Community Health*, Vol. 59.

Krieger, N. (2011) *Epidemiology and People's Health*. Oxford: Oxford University Press.

Kristof, N. (2009) "Cancer from the kitchen?" *New York Times*, December 6.

Krugman, P. (2009) "Is this the end for Harry and Louise?," *New York Times*, May 11.

Krugman, P. (2011a) "Medicare saves money," *New York Times*, June 13.

Krugman, P. (2011b) "The war on logic," *New York Times*, January 17, 2011.

Krugman, P. and Wells, R. (2006) "The health care crisis and what to do about it," *New York Review of Books*, Vol. 53, No. 5.

Landon, B. et al. (2001) "Health plan characteristics and consumers' assessments of quality," *Health Affairs*, Vol. 20, No. 2.

Lantz, P. M. et al. (1998) "Socioeconomic factors, health behaviors, and mortality: results from a nationally representative prospective study of US adults," *Journal of the American Medical Association*, Vol. 279, No. 21.

Lees, L. (1998) *The Solidarities of Strangers: The English Poor Laws and the people 1700–1948*. Cambridge: Cambridge University Press.

Leigh, J. et al. (1997) "Occupational injury and illness in the United States: estimates of costs, morbidity, and mortality," *Journal of the American Medical Association Archives of Internal Medicine*, Vol. 157, No. 14.

Leonnig, C. (2008) "U.S. rushes to change workplace toxin rules," *Washington Post*, July 23.

Lexchin, J. (1993) "Interactions between physicians and the pharmaceutical industry – what does the literature say?" *Canadian Medical Association Journal*, Vol. 149.

Light, D. W. and Lexchin, J. (2005) "Foreign free riders and the high price of US medicines," *British Medical Journal*, Vol. 331.

Lopez-Carlos, A. (2005) *The Global Competitiveness Report 2005–2006: Video interviews*. www.weforum.org/site/homepublic.nsf/Content/Global+Competitiveness+Report+2005-2006:+Interview (accessed August 12, 2006).

Lynch, J. et al. (2000) "Income inequality and mortality: importance to health of individual income, psychosocial environment, or material conditions," *British Medical Journal*, Vol. 320.

Lynch, J. et al. (2004) "Is income inequality a determinant of population health? Part 2. U.S. national and regional trends in income inequality and age- and cause-specific mortality," *Milbank Quarterly*, Vol. 82, No. 2.

MacDonald, J. and McBride, W. (2009) *The Transformation of US Livestock Agriculture: Scale, efficiency and risks*, Economic Information Bulletin no. 43, Washington DC: US Department of Agriculture Economic Research Service.

Maddison, A. (2001) *The World Economy: A millennial perspective*. Paris: OECD.

Malkan, S. (2003) "Chemical trespass: the chemical body burden and the threat to public health," *Multinational Monitor*, Vol. 24, No. 4.

Manning, W. and Marquis, M. (1996) "Health insurance: the tradeoff between risk pooling and moral hazard," *Journal of Health Economics*, Vol. 15, Issue 5.

Marmor, T. and Oberlander, J. (2010) "The health bill explained at last," *New York Review of Books*, August 19.

Marmor, T., Oberlander, J., and White, J. (2009) "The Obama administration's options for health care cost control: hope versus reality," *Annals of Internal Medicine*, Vol. 150, No. 7.

Marmot, M. (2010) *Fair Society Healthy Lives: The Marmot Review executive summary*, www.ucl.ac.uk/marmotreview (accessed June 6, 2011).

Marmot, M., Siegrist, J., and Theorell, T. (2006) "Health and the psychosocial environment at work," in M. Marmot and R. Wilkinson (eds.), *Social Determinants of Health,*. Oxford: Oxford University Press.

Marmot, M. G. and Mustard, J. F. (1994) "Coronary heart disease from a population perspective to high heart disease US," in R. G., Evans, B. L. Morris and T. R. Marmor (eds.), *Why are Some People Healthy and Others are Not?* New York: Walter de Gruyer.

Marx, K. (1967 [1867]) *Capital: Volume 1, A critical analysis of capitalist production*, (New York: International Publishers.

Mayne, L., Girod, C., and Weltz, S. (2011) *2011 Milliman Medical Index*, Milliman Research Report.

McKee-Ryan, F. et al. (2005) "Psychological and physical well-being during unemployment: a meta-analytic study," *Journal of Applied Psychology*, Vol. 90, No. 1.

McKeown, T. (1976a) *The Role of Medicine*. London: Nuffield Provincial Hospitals Trust.

McKeown, T. (1976b) *The Modern Rise of Population*. London: Edward Arnold.

McKeown, T. (1979) *The Role Of Medicine: Dream, mirage or nemesis?* 2nd edn. Oxford: Basil Blackwell.

McKeown, T. and Record, R. (1962) "Reasons for the decline of mortality in England and Wales during the nineteenth century," *Population Studies*, Vol. 16, No. 2.

McKeown, T., Record, R., and Turner, R. (1975) "An interpretation of the decline of mortality in England and Wales during the twentieth century," *Population Studies*, Vol. 29, No. 3.

McKinlay, J. and McKinlay, S. (1977) "The questionable contribution of medical measures to the decline of mortality in the United States in the twentieth century," *Milbank Memorial Fund Quarterly Health and Society*, Vol. 55, No. 3.

McKinlay, J., McKinlay, S., and Beaglehole, R. (1989) "A review of the evidence concerning the impact of medical measures on recent mortality and morbidity in the United States," *International Journal of Health Services* Vol. 19, No. 2.

McQuiston, T., Ronda, Z., and Loomis, D. (1998) "The case for stronger OSHA enforcement – evidence from evaluation research," *American Journal of Public Health*, Vol. 88, No. 7.

McWilliams, J. et al. (2007) "Health of previously uninsured adults after acquiring Medicare coverage," *Journal of the American Medical Association*, Vol. 298, No. 24.

Meeker, E. (1974) "The social rate of return on investment in public health, 1880–1910," *Journal of Economic History*, Vol. 34, No. 2.

Michaels, D. (2008) *Doubt is Their Product: How industry's assault on science threatens your health*. Oxford: Oxford University Press.

Ministry of Finance, Ontario, Canada. (2010) *Ontario's Long Term Report on the Economy*. Toronto: Queen's Printer for Ontario.

Mintzes, B. et al. (2002) "Influence of direct to consumer pharmaceutical advertising and patients' requests on prescribing decisions: two site cross sectional survey," *British Medical Journal*, Vol. 324.

Mishel, L., Bernstein, J., and Schmitt, J. (1999) *The State of Working America 1998–1999*. New York: Cornell University Press.

Mokyr, J. (1993) "Editor's introduction: the new economic history and the industrial revolution," in J. Mokyr (ed.), *The British Industrial Revolution: An economic perspective*. Boulder, Colo.: Westview Press.

Montgomery, D. (1976) "Labor in the industrial era," in R. Morris (ed.), *The American Worker*. Washington DC: US Department of Labor.

Mooney, G. (2007) "Infectious diseases and epidemiologic transition in Victorian Britain? Definitely," *Social History of Medicine*, Vol. 20, No. 3.

Mulley, A. (2009) "Inconvenient truths about supplier induced demand and unwarranted variation in medical practice," *British Medical Journal*, Vol. 339.

Muntaner, C. et al. (2004) "Economic inequality, working-class power, social capital and cause-specific mortality in wealthy countries," in V. Navarro and C. Muntaner (eds.), *Political and Economic Determinants of Population Health and Well-Being*. Amityville, N.Y.: Baywood.

Mustard, C., Lavis, J., and Ostry, A. (2006) "Work and health: new evidence and enhanced understandings," in J. Heymann et al. (eds.), *Healthier Societies: From analysis to action*. Oxford: Oxford University Press.

Nardin, R., Himmelstein, D., and Woolhandler, S. (2009) "Massachusetts is no model for national health care reform," Physicians for a National Health Program, February 20. http://pnhp.org/mass_report/mass_report_Final.pdf (accessed July 28, 2011).

National Center for Health Statistics (NCHS) (2006) *National Vital Statistics Report: Fast facts A to Z*, October. Hyattsville, Md.: NCHS.

National Coalition on Health Care (2009) *Containing Costs and Avoiding Tax Increases While Improving Quality: Affordable coverage and high value care*. http://nchc.org/blog/nchc-white-paper (accessed June 30, 2011).

National Institute for Health Care Management (NIHCM) (2002) *Changing Patterns in Pharmaceutical Innovation*. Washington DC: NIHCM.

National Institute for Occupational Safety and Health (1981) Interim Estimate.

National Nurses United (n.d.) "Nurses campaign to heal America." www. nationalnursesunited.org/pages/ncha (accessed October 11, 2012).

National Poverty Center (2010) *Poverty in the United States: Frequently asked questions*, Gerald R. Ford School of Public Policy, University of Michigan. www.npc.umich.edu/poverty (accessed February 8, 2012).

Navarro, V. (1984) "Medical history as justification rather than explanation: a critique of Starr's *The Social Transformation of American Medicine*," *International Journal of Health Services*, Vol. 14, No. 4.

Navarro, V. (1989) "Why some countries have national health insurance, others have national health services and the United States has neither," *Social Science and Medicine*, Vol. 28, No. 9.

Navarro, V. (2007) "Why Hillary's health care plan really failed," *Counterpunch*, November 12. www.counterpunch.org/2007/11/12/why-hillary-s-health-care-plan-really-failed (accessed September 21, 2011).

Navarro, V. et al. (2003) "The importance of the political and the social in explaining mortality differentials amongst countries of the OECD, 1950–1998," *International Journal of Health Services*, Vol. 33, No. 3.

Navarro, V. et al. (2004) "Summary and conclusions of the study," in V. Navarro (ed.), *The Political and Social Contests of Health*. Amityville, N.Y.: Baywood.

Neergaard, L. (2011) "Government announces plan to reduce health disparities," *American Press*, April 8, www.physorg.com/news/2011-04-govt-health-disparities.html (accessed August 3, 2011).

Nettle, D. (2010) "Why are there social gradients in preventative health behavior? A perspective from behavioral ecology," *PLoS ONE*, Vol. 5, No. 10.

New York Times (1910) "Soothing syrups," *New York Times*, August 30.

Newhouse, J. (1993) *Free For All?: Lessons From the Rand health insurance experiment*. Cambridge, Mass.: Harvard University Press.

Nyman, J. (2003) *The Theory of Demand for Health Insurance*. Stanford, Calif.: Stanford University Press.

Oakes, L. and Norfleet, N. (2012) "Today's special: Moorhead waitress gets her $12,000 tip," *StarTribune*, April 5. www.startribune.com/local/146315905.html (accessed April 6, 2012).

Offer, A., Pechey, R., and Ulijaszek, S. (2010) "Obesity under affluence varies by welfare regimes: the effect of fast food, insecurity, and inequality," *Economics and Human Biology,* Vol. 6, No. 3.

Okun, A. (1975) *Equality and Efficiency: The big tradeoff.* Washington DC: Brookings Institution.

Oliver, A. (2007) The Veterans Health Administration: an American success story?," *Milbank Quarterly,* Vol. 85, No. 1.

Olsen, G. (2011). *Power and Inequality: A comparative introduction.* Oxford: Oxford University Press.

Ontario Ministry of Health and Long Term Care. (2010) *Ontario Wait Times: Wait times for surgery, MRIs and CTs.* www.waittimes.net/Surgerydi/en/PublicMain.aspx?Type=0 (accessed March 1, 2012).

OECD (2002) *Health Data 2002.* Paris: OECD.

OECD (2010) *OECD Health Data 2010.* www.oecd.org/health/healthdata (accessed March 21, 2011).

OECD (2011) *Health at a Glance 2011: OECD Indicators,* http://dx.doi.org/10.1787/health_glance-2011-en (accessed April 3, 2012).

Osborne, A. (2003) "2m jobs 'at risk' in chemicals sector," *Guardian,* July 15. www.guardian.co.uk/business/2003/jul/15/environment.conservation (accessed August 5, 2011).

Ouyang, X. et al. (2008) "Fructose consumption as a risk factor for non-alcoholic fatty liver disease," *Journal of Hepatology,* Vol. 48, No. 6.

Palmer, B. (1983) *Working-Class Experience.* Toronto: Butterworths Canada.

Pauly, M. (1968) "The economics of moral hazard: comment," *American Economic Review,* Vol. 58, No. 3.

PBS (1998) *America 1900: The Idle Rich,* www.pbs.org/wgbh/amex/1900/peopleevents/pande28.html (accessed April 6, 2012).

PBS (2000) *American Experience: The Rockefellers,* www.pbs.org/wgbh/amex/rockefellers/sfeature/sf_8.html (accessed April 12, 2011).

PBS (2007) *Ghost in Your Genes.* www.pbs.org/wgbh/nova/genes/expert.html (accessed March 31, 2011).

Pear, R. (2009) "Doctors' group opposes public insurance plan," *New York Times,* June 11.

Pearce, N. (2008) "Corporate influences on epidemiology," *International Journal of Epidemiology,* Vol. 37, No. 1.

Pessen, E. (1976) "Builders of the young republic," in R. Morris (ed.), *The American Worker.* Washington DC: US Department of Labor.

Peterson, C. and Burton, R. (2007) *US Health Care Spending: Comparison with other OECD countries.* Washington DC: Congressional Research Service.

Physicians for a National Health Program. (n.d.) "Single-payer national health insurance." www.pnhp.org/facts/single-payer-resources (accessed October 11, 2012).

Picard, A. (2005) "Our health care serves up profits," *Globe and Mail,* December 1.

Piketty, T. and Saez, E. (2003) "Income inequality in the United States, 1913–1998," *Quarterly Journal of Economics,* Vol. 118, No. 1.

Poland, B et al. (1998) "Wealth, equality and health care: a critique of a 'population health' perspective on the determinants of health," *Social Science and Medicine* Vol. 46, No. 7.

Polanyi, K. (1944) *The Great Transformation*. Boston, Mass.: Beacon Press.

Pollack, A. (2003a) "Tenet Healthcare reports $55 million quarterly loss," *New York Times*, April 11.

Pollack, A. (2003b) "Tenet reports new investigation of its deal with doctors," *New York Times*, July 16.

Pollan, M. (2002a) "Power steer," *New York Times Magazine*, March 31.

Pollan, M. (2002b) "When a crop becomes king," *New York Times*, July 19.

Pollin, R. (2003) *Contours of Descent: US economic fractures and the landscape of global austerity*. London: Verso.

Porter, D. (1999) *Health, Civilization and the State: A history of public health from ancient to modern times*. New York: Routledge.

Porter, J., Ogden, J., and Pronyk, P. (1999) "Infectious disease policy: towards the production of health," *Health Policy and Planning* Vol. 14, No. 4.

Porter, M. (2000) "Location, competition, and economic development: local clusters in a global economy," *Economic Development Quarterly*, Vol. 14, No. 1.

Potter, W. (2010) *Deadly Spin*. London: Bloomsbury.

Public Citizen Health Research Group (1985) *Dyes in Your Food*. www.feingold.org/Research/dyesinfood.html (accessed August 13, 2011).

Quadagno, J. (2004) "Why the United States has no national health insurance: stakeholder mobilization against the welfare state, 1945–1996," *Journal of Health and Social Behavior*, Vol. 45, extra issue.

Rachlis, M. (2004) *Prescription for Excellence: How innovation is saving Canada's health care system*. Toronto: HarperCollins.

Rachlis, R. and Kushner, K. (1989) *Second Opinion*. Toronto: HarperCollins.

Raff, D. (1988) "Wage determination theory and the five-dollar day at Ford," *Journal of Economic History*, Vol. 48, No. 2.

Randall, V. (2002) "Racial discrimination in health care in the United States as a violation of the International Convention on the Elimination of All Forms of Racial Discrimination," *University of Florida Journal of Law and Public Policy*, Vol. 45.

Raphael, D. (2003). "A society in decline: the social, economic, and political determinants of health inequalities in the USA," in R. Hofrichter (ed.), *Health and Social Justice: A reader on politics, ideology, and inequity in the distribution of disease*. San Francisco, Calif.: Jossey Bass/Wiley.

Raphael, D. (2010) "Social determinants of health: an overview of key issues and themes," in L. Fernandez, S. MacKinnon, and J. Silver (eds.), *The Social Determinants of Health in Manitoba,*. Winnipeg, MB: CCBA-MB.

Raphael, D. and Bryant, T. (2004) "The welfare state as a determinant of women's health: support for omen's quality of life in Canada and four comparison nations," *Health Policy*, Vol. 68, No. 1.

Reagan, R. (1974) "We will be a city upon a hill," January 25. First Conservative Political Action Conference, http://reagan2020.us/speeches/City_Upon_A_Hill.asp (accessed April 6, 2012).

Reich, R. (2010) *Aftershock: The next economy and America's future*. New York: Knopf.

Relman, A. (1980) "The new medical–industrial complex," *New England Journal of Medicine*, Vol. 303, No. 17.

Reinier, K. et al. (2011) "Socioeconomic status and incidence of sudden cardiac arrest," *Canadian Medical Association Journal*, Vol. 183, No. 15.

Reuben, S. (2010) *Reducing Environmental Cancer Risk: President's Cancer Panel 2008–2009*. Washington DC: US Department of Health and Human Services.

Rogot, E. et al. (1992) *A Mortality Study of 1.3 million persons*. Bethesda, Md.: National Institutes of Health, National Heart, Lung and Blood Institute.

Rose, G. and Marmot, M.G. (1981) "Social class and coronary heart disease," *British Heart Journal*, Vol. 45, No. 1.

Rosen, G. (1958) *A History of Public Health*. New York: MD Publications.

Rosenbloom, J. and Stutes, G. (2008) "Reexamining the distribution of wealth in 1870," in J. Rosenbloom (ed.), *Quantitative Economic History: The good of counting*. New York: Routledge.

Rosner, D. and Markowitz, G. (1997) "The early movement for occupational safety and health," in J. Leavitt and R. Numbers (eds.), *Sickness and Health in America*. Madison, Wisc.: University of Wisconsin Press.

Ross, N. et al. (2006) "Income inequality as a determinant of health," in J. Heymann, C. Hertzman, M. Barer and R. Evans (eds.), *Healthier Societies: From analysis to action*. Oxford: Oxford University Press.

Rust, S. (2008) "FDA relied on industry studies to judge safety," *Milwaukee Journal Sentinel*, March 21.

Sachs, N. (2009) "Jumping the pond: transnational law and the future of chemical regulation," *Vanderbilt Law Review*, Vol. 62, No. 6.

Sager, A. and Socolar, D. (2005) *Health Costs Absorb One-Quarter of Economic Growth, 2000–2005*, Data Brief no. 8–9 February. Boston, Mass.: Boston University School of Public Health.

Sargent, M. (2005) *Biomedicine and the Human Condition: Challenges, risks and rewards*. Cambridge: Cambridge University Press.

Satcher, D. and Higginbotham, E. (2008) "The public health approach to eliminating disparities in health," *American Journal of Public Health*, Vol. 98, No. 3.

Schlaff, A. (2008) "Satcher and Higginbotham: NOT the public health response," *American Journal of Public Health,* Vol. 98. No. 3.

Schoen, C., Collins, S., and Kriss, J. (2008): "How many are underinsured? Trends among U.S. adults, 2003 and 2007," *Health Affairs,* June.

Schoen, C. et al. (2005) "Taking the pulse of health care systems: experiences of patients with health problems in six countries," *Health Affairs* web exclusive.

Schwab, K. (2010) *The Global Competitiveness Report 2010–2011.* Geneva: World Economic Forum.

Seaton, A. (2000) "Occupational lung diseases," in A. Seaton et al. (eds.), *Crofton and Douglas's Respiratory Diseases, Vol. 2,* 5th edn. Malden, Mass.: Blackwell Science.

Sepehri, A. and Chernomas, R. (2004) "Is the Canadian health care system fiscally sustainable?" *International Journal of Health Services,* Vol. 34, No. 2.

Shaffer, E. and Brenner, J. (2004) "Trade and health care: corporatizing vital human services," in M. Fort, M-A. Mercer, and O. Gish (eds.), *Sickness and Health: The corporate assault on global health.* Cambridge, Mass.: South End Press.

Shafrin, J. (2010) "Operating on commission: analyzing how physician financial incentives affect surgery rates," *Health Economics,* Vol. 19, No. 5.

Shaikh, A. (1986) "Exploitation," in J. Eatwell, M. Milgate, and P. Newman (eds.), *The New Palgrave: A dictionary of economic theory and doctrine.* London: Macmillan.

Shaikh, A. (2011) "The first great depression of the 21st century," in G. Albo, V. Chibber, and L. Panitch (eds.), *Socialist Register 2011: The crisis this time, Vol. 47.* New York: Monthly Review Press.

Shen, Y. C. (2002) "The effect of hospital ownership choice on patient outcomes after treatment for acute myocardial infarction," *Journal of Health Economics,* Vol. 21, Issue 5.

Shoham, D. et al. (2008) "Sugary soda consumption and albuminuria: results from the National Health and Nutrition Examination Survey, 1999–2004," *PLoS One,* Vol. 3, No. 10.

Silverman, E., Skinner, J., and Fischer, E. (1999) "The association between for-profit hospital ownership and increased Medicare spending," *New England Journal of Medicine,* Vol. 341, No. 6.

Singer, N. (2009) "Harry and Louise return, with a new message," *New York Times,* July 16.

Singh, G. and Siahpush, M. (2006) "Widening socioeconomic inequalities in US life expectancy, 1980–2000," *International Journal of Epidemiology,* Vol. 35. No. 4.

Sirovich, B. et al. (2008) "Discretionary decision making by primary care physicians and the cost of U.S. Health care," *Health Affairs* Vol. 27, No. 3.

Skinner, J. and Fisher, E. (2010) "The Dartmouth team responds – again – to Ms. Abelson and Mr. Harris of the *New York Times,*" *New York Times,* June 22.

Sparer, M. (2009) "Health care 2009: Medicaid and the U.S. path to national health insurance," *New England Journal of Medicine,* Vol. 360, No. 4.

Starr, P. (1982) *The Social Transformation of American Medicine.* New York: Basic Books.

Stiglitz, J. (2011) "Of the 1%, by the 1%, for the 1%," *Vanity Fair*, May.

Stolberg, S. and Gerth, J. (2000) "High-tech stealth being used to sway doctor prescriptions," *New York Times*, Nov. 16.

Szreter, S. (1988) "The importance of social intervention in Britain's mortality decline 1850–1914: a reinterpretation of the role of public health," *Social History of Medicine*, Vol. 1, No. 1.

Szreter, S. (2002a) "Rethinking McKeown: the relationship between public health and social change," *American Journal of Public Health*, Vol. 92, No. 5.

Szreter, S. (2002b) "The state of social capital: bringing back in power, politics, and history," *Theory and Society*, Vol. 31, No. 5.

Szreter, S. (2003) "The population health approach in historical perspective," *American Journal of Public Health*, Vol. 93, No. 2.

Szreter, S. (2004a) "Industrialization and health," *British Medical Bulletin*, Vol. 69.

Szreter, S. (2004b) "Author response: debating mortality trends in 19th century Britain," *International Journal of Epidemiology*, Vol. 33, No. 4.

Thurow, L. (1996) *The Future of Capitalism: How today's economic forces shape tomorrow's world*. New York: Penguin.

Tomasky, M. (2010) "The money fighting health care reform," *New York Review of Books*, April 8, Vol. 17, No. 6.

Trasande, L. and Liu, Y. (2011) "Reducing the staggering costs of environmental disease in children, estimated at $76.6 billion in 2008," *Health Affairs*, Vol. 30, No. 5.

Union of Concerned Scientists (2008) *Interference at the EPA: Science and politics at the US Environmental Protection Agency*. Cambridge, Mass.: Union of Concerned Scientists.

United Nations (2011) *UN International Human Development Indicators*, http://hdr.undp.org/en/data/ (accessed March 15, 2011).

US Administration on Aging (2010) "Projected future growth of the older population," www.aoa.gov/aoaroo/aging_statistics/future_growth/future_growth.aspx#age (accessed May 6, 2011).

US Department of Health and Education, and Welfare (1977) *Occupational Diseases*. Washington D.C.: US Government Printing Office.

US Department of Health and Human Services (2010) *Update on Bisphenol A (BPA) for Use in Food: January 2010*, www.fda.gov/newsevents/publichealthfocus/ucm064437.htm (accessed May 31, 2011).

US National Institute of Health (2009) "Exploring the roles of cancer centers for integrating aging and cancer research," www.nia.nih.gov/ResearchInformation/ConferencesAndMeetings/WorkshopReport/Figure1.htm (accessed May 6, 2011).

Vaillancourt, R. and Linder, S. (2003) "Two decades of research comparing for-profit and nonprofit health provider performance in the United States," *Social Science Quarterly*, Vol. 84, No. 2.

Von Tunzelmann, N. (1994) "Technology in the early nineteenth century," in R. Floud and D. N. McCloskey (eds.), *The Economic History of Britain Since 1700*, 2nd edn. Cambridge: Cambridge University Press.

Voth, H. (2003) "Living standards during the industrial revolution: an economists' guide," *American Economic Review*, Vol. 93, No. 2.

Waitzkin, H. (2011) *Medicine and Public Health at the End of Empire*. Boulder, Colo.: Paradigm.

Waldbott , G. (1978) Health Effects of Environmental Pollutants, St Louis, Miss.: C.V. Mosby.

Walker, E. (2010) "Health insurers post record profits," *ABC News*. http://abcnews.go.com/Health/HealthCare/health-insurers-post-record-profits/story?id=9818699 (accessed July 20, 2011).

Walker, P. et al. (2005) "Public health implications of meat production and consumption," *Public Health Nutrition*, Vol. 8, No. 4.

Weil, D. (1996) "If OSHA is so bad, why is compliance so good?," *RAND Journal of Economics*, Vol. 27, No. 3.

Weinstein, J. (1968) *The Corporate Ideal in the Liberal State 1900-1918*. Boston, Mass.: Beacon Press.

Whaples, R. (2010) "Hours of work in US history," EH.net, http://eh.net/encyclopedia/article/whaples.work.hours.us (accessed April 6, 2011).

White, M. (1991). *Against Unemployment*. London: PSI.

Wilkinson, R. (1996) *Unhealthy Societies*. London: Routledge.

Wilkinson, R. and Pickett, K. (2009) *The Spirit Level: Why more equal societies almost always do better*. New York: Bloomsbury.

Willey, J., Sherwood, L., and Woolverton, C. (2010) *Prescott's Microbiology*, 8th edn. New York: McGraw-Hill.

Williams, D., Lavizzo-Mourey, R., and Warren, R. (1994) "The concept of race and health status in America," *Public Health Reports*, Vol. 109, No. 1.

Williamson, J. (1994) "Coping with city growth," in R. Floud and D. McCloskey (eds.), *The Economic History of Britain Since 1700*, 2nd edn. Cambridge: Cambridge University Press.

Wolff, L. (1965) *Lockout: The story of the homestead strike of 1892*. London: Longmans.

Woolf, S. (2011) "Public health implications of government spending reductions," *Journal of the American Medical Association*, Vol. 305, No. 18.

Woolhandler, S., Campbell, T., and Himmelstein, D. (2003) "Costs of health care administration in the United States and Canada," *New England Journal of Medicine*, Vol. 349, No. 8.

Woolhandler, S. and Himmelstein, D. (1997) "Costs of care and administration at for-profit and other hospitals in the United States," *New England Journal of Medicine*, Vol. 336, No. 11.

Woolhandler, S. and Himmelstein, D. (2007a) "Competition in a publicly funded healthcare system," *British Medical Journal*, Vol. 335.

Woolhandler, S. and Himmelstein, D. (2007b) "Health reform failure," *Boston Globe*, September 17.

World Health Organization (WHO) (2008a) "Inequities are killing people on grand scale," press release, August 28, www.who.int/mediacentre/news/releases/2008/pr29/en/index.html (accessed August 3, 2011).

WHO (2008b) *WHO Commission on the Social Determinants of Health.* Geneva, WHO.

WHO (2010) *Tuberculosis,* fact sheet no. 104. Geneva, WHO.

Wrigley, E. and Schofield, R. (1981) *The Population History of England 1541–1871: A reconstruction.* Cambridge: Cambridge University Press.

Ziegler, R. G. *et al.* (1993) "Migration patterns and breast cancer risk in Asian-American women," *Journal of the National Cancer Institute,* Vol. 85, No. 22.

Zipkin, D. and Steinman, M. (2005) "Interactions between pharmaceutical representatives and doctors in training: a thematic review," *Journal of General Internal Medicine,* Vol. 20, No. 8.

Zweig, M. (2000) *The Working Class Majority: America's best kept secret.* Ithaca, N.Y.: Cornell University Press.

INDEX